THE POWER GURU OF MONSTA GARAGE

How Dan Fa'asamala's Methods Make Men into Bench Pressing Monstas

by

Eric Burtson

Table of Contents

Foreword by Joe Schmidt
Introduction
Part I: Guru and Garage
Chapter 1. Monsta Garage: "Do you really wanna be that strong?"
Chapter 2. The Making of a Guru: Learning
Chapter 3. The Making of a Guru: Mastering
Part II: Guru's Practice
Chapter 4. Technique
Chapter 5. Motivation and Consistency
Chapter 6. Guru Coaching
Chapter 7. Heart
Epilogue

Copyright 2014 Eric Burtson

ALL RIGHTS RESERVED

No part of this publication may be reproduced in any form or my any means — electronic, mechanical, photocopy, recording or otherwise — without prior written permission, except for the inclusion of brief quotations in a review.

Cover design by C. Michael Pedersen

ISBN: 978-0-9909287-1-3

To Roger Metz, the Guru's guru.

FOREWORD BY JOE SCHMIDT

It was mid July of 2013 when I was first introduced to the "product" of Dan's Monsta Garage and his famous medium-wide suicide grip. Eric Burtson, the author of this book, former boss and colleague and current good friend, had agreed to meet me for a beer at the South Park Abbey. It had been at least six weeks since the last time I saw Eric, and something looked different about him. He was walking towards me with his normal enthusiastic gait, a smile from ear to ear, and a friendly hand outstretched in search of another to shake. When we shook, that's when I saw it. By nature, Eric is a lean man, looking more like Dr. Drew than Arnold Schwarzenegger. But on this day his bulging triceps made him look more like an over-the-hill Abercrombie and Fitch model than Bill Nye the Science Guy.

Beers were drunk and a conversation that would change my life ensued. I've never been an athlete and the only thing I ever lifted with any frequency was a California Burrito around two o'clock in the morning. That didn't stop Eric from filling my head with details about this guy named Dan and his specialized lifting techniques. Much of the information Eric shared that afternoon was lost on me. At that time I didn't understand the technicalities or anything about the world of competitive strength lifting. But there were two things I understood completely from that first conversation: the fevered excitement in Eric's voice while he told me about "the best gym in the world" and those triceps. I was sold.

The following Friday, I made the hour-long trek with Eric and his son Alex, from San Diego to an average suburban garage in Oceanside where everything but the average was happening. That night I met the Guru, took to his bench and never looked back. I've been going to Dan's with Eric and his family for slightly over a year. I've learned a lot about power lifting, and all those technicalities Eric was telling me about at the Abbey started to make sense. It was working; I was getting stronger.

A year later, I'm stronger in my upper body then I've ever been in my life. As the author of this book describes, I did suffer from a "weekend jackhammer accident". I assure you, there is no double entendre intended in that statement. I was helping a friend bust up a cement foundation with a jackhammer and I injured my left arm, inhibiting my progress for nine long months. Eventually my injury healed and my progress resumed. Not too long ago, I was shocked to see myself pushing 235 pounds! I only did it once and it wasn't pretty, but I did it. For a guy that struggled to push the 55-pound bar on his first night, this was pretty epic.

Dan Fa'asamala, "The Guru" is a remarkable man with an amazing gift. Dan has the ability to inspire one's heart. From my perspective, he's a soft-spoken sage who exudes patience, wisdom, and generosity. Some men are leaders because they have been trained to be. Some men are leaders because circumstances force them to be. And some men, like Dan, are leaders because their heart won't let them be anything else. There is something about the man that brings out the best in people. Dan Fa'asamala is able to push people beyond their own expectations. When he sizes you up for the first time, you can't help but feel like he knows your capabilities better than you do. I think what it comes down to is this: Dan knows heart. And Dan knows how to build heart.

Over the past year, It has been my privilege to get to know Eric Burtson, his wife Paige, his son Alex, his daughter Cherish, and his youngest son Jonny. Eric is an accomplished and successful man. You can tell this by the relationship he has with his family, and they with each other. There is a candor and quirky humor they share that is both remarkable and inspiring. Personally, this last year has been devastating to my family and me. Internal dynamics went all wrong, and it left me in a funk. Eric Burtson opened his home, family, and his amazing friendship with Dan Fa'asamala to me. This helped bring light to my darkness. There is a common thread of generosity that binds Dan and his Monsta Garage to the Burtson family. These are people who give from the heart to build you up. These are people who know that the secret to power is heart.

INTRODUCTION

Daniel Fa'asamala had a strong start in sports. He was a football standout, a wrestling champion and a contender in the Natural Teenage Mr. America. But after he graduated from high school that was all behind him. He turned down a wrestling scholarship so he could watch over his family.

With nothing else to do, he started lifting in his garage, leaving the door open. People started coming by to lift. Eventually his sons lifted with him. Then their friends came. Dan's Monsta Garage had no formal memberships, no money changing hands, and no recruiting, yet it went on to produce four champions breaking five world records in the AAU drug-free bench-press competitions.

This book is about the Monsta-building lifting techniques and coaching approaches Dan Fa'asamala developed over decades of trial and error in his Monsta Garage. If you are a lifter looking to get stronger, this book is for you. If you are a gym owner, personal trainer, or coach, this book will help you take the next steps on the way to guru status.

Chapter 1 is an overview of what Monsta Gym looks like.

Chapter 2 gives insight into the development of a special person in tenacious pursuit of physical power.

Chapter 3 shows the environment in which the Guru was able to focus his knowledge toward the development of power in other people.

Chapter 4, *Technique*, explains the unique lifting style in detail.

Chapter 5, *Motivation and Consistency*, is likely the most important chapter because it explains how to keep people coming back to lift on a regular basis. Without consistency, there can be no gains.

Chapter 6, *Guru Coaching*, shows the importance of a guru to achieve the highest levels of muscular development. After reading this, you will see how Dan distinguishes himself above the typical gym owner or personal trainer.

Chapter 7, *Heart*, is about what distinguishes you, what propels you to the realm of the impossible.

Part I: GURU AND GARAGE

1. Monsta Garage

Do you really wanna be that strong?

FIRST EXPEDITION

Though Dan Fa'asamala has been training men in his garage from the early 1980's, it wasn't until the new millennium approached that someone finally asked, "Hey, why don't we see how we do in a real competition?" So, in 1999 Jason Padgette represented Monsta gym in the 181 lb., 16-17 year-old division, and just like that, they had their first AAU drug-free bench-press American record holder. Over the next four years, Danny and his lifters broke five world bench press records in a shocking display of power — possibly unprecedented for a gym so small.

How did he do it? How did they do it? There to witness these achievements was the AAU's Assistant National Chairman for all strength sports, Martin Drake. When I asked him what he wanted to say about Dan Fa'asamala, Martin replied, "Dan Fa'asamala is a mover and shaker of lives."

Martin was impressed enough by Dan and his gym that he nominated Dan for the AAU North American Powerlifting Hall of Fame award, which Dan did receive. To be fair, Martin was most impressed with Dan's affect on people's motivation than anything else. Martin went on to say, "Dan is a master of getting people to get the most out of themselves through relationship."

In these two statements Martin connected to the reasons for this book: first, to document how it is possible to nurture so much muscle-power in so few individuals, and second, how one man can deeply motivate others through positive intention, knowledgeable oversight, and power of the personality.

THE GYM TODAY

"I'm going to the best gym on the planet," I told myself out loud on the drive from San Diego to Oceanside. I repeated it, not as some sort of psyche-up ritual, but to punctuate the reality of the situation—that, despite the availability of the gym, I had never gone. I was amazed at myself for having taken so long to take up my best friend's offer to lift at what I told myself was the best gym on the planet. Ridiculous. It had been thirty years since Dan invited me up. It had been fifteen years since he started producing world champions, and finally, I was going.

It's not like I don't care about lifting. Dan and I started on the weights in high school. I was a sophomore, and Dan was a freshman at Carlsbad High, 1977. We both played football, and somehow I talked him into joining the wrestling team. Our bodies responded to the workouts, and we quickly realized that to get better than the rest we had to work out harder than the rest. Since we weren't joggers, our best investment would be in muscle.

The problem was that in 1977 high school gyms looked more like a Motel-6 workout area: a few plastic mats and a single carousel of weight equipment, those push-pin levered lifting machines. We knew that wouldn't cut it, so we got in Dan's car—yes, without a driver's license—and found Iron Man's Gym in Oceanside. That's where the education began; that was the foundation for the "best gym on the planet". More on that later.

It was Monday, May 20, 2013 and I was driving up I5. What is "best" anyway? Best depends, of course, on what you are measuring. Best money-maker? No, Monsta Gym is not incorporated. It's just Dan's garage. Best Olympic lifters? Nope. No clean-and-jerk at Monsta. Best body-builder's gym? Not that either. Dan placed 5th in the Teenage Mr. America back when he was in high school, but what goes on at Monsta Gym now has nothing at all to do with cutting weight.

Monsta Gym is most like a power lifting gym, just without the deadlift and squat. It's all about the bench press, and it's all about power. This creates some controversy, because it seems unbalanced. But, as I found out, Monsta Gym is very much focused on the functionality of the power acquired through its methods.

Dan's Monsta gym has cracked the code on creating upper body strength, and it does this strictly without the help of steroids. Monsta Gym has done so much with so little. It has never had a push for members. Whoever shows up in the garage gets to lift, free. There are no franchises, no multiple sessions, just a few guys at a Monday and a Friday night workout. Yet it has four individuals holding five world titles in AAU bench-press.

Being drug free is obviously important to my claim. Without it, we cannot say Monsta's process is what works. Incidentally, some of the records come close to the records held in un-drug-tested venues. And some beat these anyway.

Some people have made the claim that Monsta is boosted by being in Oceanside, fed by the surrounding Samoan community. Oceanside brought us Junior Seau. In fact, Dan Fa'asamala is Samoan. But if you are among those who believe Samoans are stronger than your average mortal, know this: most Monstas are not Samoan; one of its world record holders is African American; and another is white; another is half-Samoan.

After driving East on the 78, I turned north up College Blvd, winding my way to Dan's garage-full of monsters. It was 7:30 in the evening. People trickled in, greeting one another with hugs. Soon Dan yelled, "Stretch! Four minutes!" I followed what everyone else did, making windmills with my arms and finding some piece of equipment on which to hitch my hands behind my back.

In life outside the gym, whenever Dan wore a suit, he looked like the Marvel super-villain "The Kingpin," massive arms and chest in a tailored suit, looking like he could pick you up by the neck with one hand and move you around like a chess piece. Well, he actually could do that. That night he was in a Monsta shirt.

Besides Dan, here is who was there on that first day: Big John, a quiet but huge man. He was Samoan. Then there was Derrick, a lean African-American man. Jonathan was also there with his friend Jarrad. They played in a band together, some sort of combination death metal and reggae-ska. Or maybe their style depended on the venue, I forget. Jonathan was a tall, muscular blond haired youth who looked like an all-American linebacker (or the model for the Bob's Big Boy statue, but more athletic looking). Jarrad looked like a skateboarding musician. Both were white.

Then there was Pete. At first, I didn't know if Pete was Mid-Eastern or Hispanic. Pete was strong, but not the strongest. He looked the most impressive though. He was 6-foot-four. Any way you looked at his upper body, it was THICK. From the side it was thick. Face-on it was thick. And Pete's arms were huge, as if someone felled a giant teak tree, put it on a lathe, and made foundation columns for someone's palace, until Pete took them for himself.

Zeke came too. He was Pete's little brother (maybe not by age, but definitely by size). Zeke was new, and didn't lift much yet. But he was fun and fun loving. He seemed to be the most excited to get started.

Finally there was me, a Polish-Italian-Norwegian transplant from the East Coast.

This demographic profile, witnessed there on day one, never shifted much from that mix over the next year of my attendance: four or five races, ages ranging from 20 to 50, body mass from 150 up to 400 lbs., and a lifting weight starting at a count of one plate on each side and going up from there, way up.

There was one bench in the garage, a big steel foundation holding a dead-lift bar, 10 pounds heavier than a normal bench bar. The extra metal kept the bar from bouncing and flexing so much when it gets loaded up. Behind the bench was a wall-sized set of shelves, holding typical household items, plus a few basketball-sized green hulk fists, and most importantly, right in the center, halfway between the ears of the bench presser and his spotter, was a giant boom box. Appropriately for this gym, the bass was boosted.

After the stretch, the workout started with Dan twisting around to press play. The first song began with the sound of footsteps, "Dead man walking". The music started, "Rollin' rollin' rollin'!" Throughout the workout the music played. It was loud. It motivated. Dan's son Beau helped make the mix, which included anything from Limp Bizkit to 80's House music.

Dan started off the workout. He was, as always, the main spotter. He stood behind the bar all night, except when he lifted. Dan went first, and Pete spotted him. After that, it was Pete's turn. Pete was barefoot. He got on the bench, and then curled up so that his feet were completely off the ground, dangling above the foot of the bench. Pete was probably the best example of the Guru's disciple, observing the lifting form to the letter of the law. Not everyone raised the feet. But everyone followed the rest of the rules.

First, the grip—in Monsta Garage lifters grip the bar with a hand separation that is halfway between conventional bench and what's called the "close grip". Then, the hold is further modified via the "suicide grip," so titled because the thumb is not permitted to wrap around the bar, as it usually does. Instead, only the inside of the wrist prevents the bar from sliding down and smashing the lifter.

Next, the lift itself starts at a particular line on the chest and ends before completion, with the lower and upper arms never going fully straight. There is no pause at the top. When some lifters try to bring it back down quickly for the next rep, Dan reminds them during the lift to just let it come down naturally, no jerking.

Finally, the set ends when the lifter can lift no more, or, when the lifter has attained his working weight range, after the spotter has assisted with a rep or two.

Pete did all that perfectly as he always does, but being the devotee he is, he continued the practice Dan used to teach long ago—that the lifter watch the bar all the way up and all the way down. This resulted in an eerie effect. We could see Pete's eyes go up and down following the bar on its journey. He even brought his head up to watch, like a dying man studying his heart monitor.

As big as Pete was, he—like all of us—started off with only two plates, one on each side, 145 lbs. When he finished his first set, we each took a turn, in a hierarchy called out by the Guru himself. Dan arranged the lifters from strongest to weakest. He did this, I learned later, for two reasons: one, out of convenience, and two, to motivate people to move up in ranks.

We stayed at this low warm-up weight for another set. Then Dan put on a 25 and had Pete put one on the other end. We did more sets. Then, they took off the 25 and put on another 45. Halfway through the roster, they took off the plate and replaced the 25 for those at the end of the rankings who could not yet lift 235 lbs. This was the start of the separation and the beginning of the personalization for each lifter for the night.

I commented to Derrick, "They don't believe in 10-pound plates at this gym."

"No 35's either," he said. And that was true all night long. Those increments are too small. Adjusting by 25s on each side, that's up or down 50 pounds at a time. I guess using the 10s at Monsta Gym would be like an NFL lineman weighing his food on a gram scale. It ain't gonna happen.

The weights just got bigger and bigger for the guys on the upper end. I don't remember if they stopped at three plates and a 25, or if Dan and John went to four or more plates, but I do remember that characteristic sound of stacks of plates jostling like a cluster of muted bells—Monsta chimes. On the next workout I would see Jason Padgette rep with five plates and I would hear the chimes again.

This is where the workout got intense. And that's when the Guru started his real coaching. During the lift I heard, "Do you really wanna be that strong?!" or as someone stretched out under the bar to start a lift he said "This is for you; you're the only one under that bar," to another person he said "Get a good feel".

Derrick came off the bench reciting words of the song that was just playing: "If you wanna move something, you gotta move it with your mind!"

After staying in each person's hard-working range, Dan took some people one plate higher, where a "monsta" could maybe get just one rep or one rep with assistance.

Then he reversed the workout taking off weights until we were back near the starting weight.

He told us this was a light night. Friday would be the heavy day.

After the workout, a few people lingered. Dan gave me a debriefing, since this was my first time at Monsta Gym.

I told him my goal was to do 300 lbs again, as I did when I was 24. Soon after I had gotten 300 that last time, I gave up lifting, picking it up again fifteen years later when my son Alex turned 14. Dan said I would get 300 again, no problem.

Dan told me about Derrick's goal when he came the first time. He wanted to do 200. Six months later—that night—he was repping 235.

Dan also told a story about Pete—how Pete originally came as an observer, and a very skinny one at that. Dan said:

> Pete showed up to the garage every day, just to be there. I used to watch him, and he was one of Beau's best friends. I said, ok, he's not in the way, he's just watching and supporting, whatever.
>
> Then one night Beau came to me and said, *"Hey Pops, is it ok if Peter joins us or lifts with us?"*
>
> *Ya, he might as well, he's there anyways — what the heck?*

My first night ended with anticipation for the next workout. As we did upon arrival, we hugged, and then left.

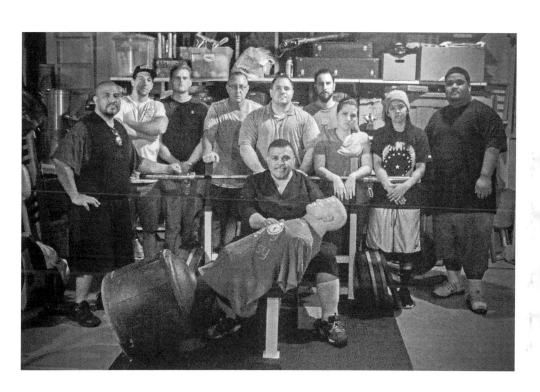

2. The Making of a Guru: Learning

MEETING

Dan and I grew up on top of a hill South of the 78 Freeway in the Tri-City region of Northern San Diego County. My backyard fence on Vista Calaveras Street marked the border with Carlsbad. Dan lived on Alto Street, one block over and halfway down the hill. He would often sit in his garage.

Dan's father, Liamatua, was a spiritual man. He would read the Bible every day to his children, Dan, Mavis, Betty, Eddie and Sam. Dan would tell is Father, "Daddy, when I grow up I want to be strong as Samson."

I met Dan with him probably thinking he was Samson. Unfortunately for me, I was the Philistine of fifth grade. Kevin Kampley was my friend and the neighborhood fight promoter. He told Dan there was this guy on Vista Calaveras Street who said he could beat up anybody.

Kevin was talking about me. I was anything but a bully. But I was big for my age, so things were set in motion. Dan challenged me to a fight. It was supposed to happen at school. Instead it happened at the bus stop at the top of the hill, somewhere between both our houses.

Before I knew it I was on the ground, and Mrs. Daniels, a true local saint, came running at us saying, "Eric Burtson, leave that poor Samoan boy alone!" She must have been going blind by then, because I was not winning.

The next time I saw Dan I was walking down Alto Street. He was sitting in his garage. We started talking about comic books. B Dan said he had been in the back of the Alpha-Beta in Carlsbad when he saw a guy unloading comics from a truck. It was Stan Lee, owner of Marvel Comics! I was amazed. We talked about comic books for three hours. Dan's favorite, of course, was the Incredible Hulk.

DISCOVERING WEIGHTS

Between the two of us, I was the first person to get interested in weights, probably because Dan was still in Middle School my freshman year at Carlsbad High.

Each Friday, my PE coach would have a weight lifting tournament among all 50 of us boys. Half were freshmen, the other half were sophomores. During that very first tournament, people started encouraging me. I was one of the survivors representing the freshmen, so even those who dropped out of the lift-off had a personal interest. It was strange to me to get any athletic acknowledgment since I spent most of my school life as an overweight nerd. By high school I had leaned down, and had played sports each season, but I hadn't excelled, until maybe now.

The tournament pressed on, each person taking turns at one of the two bench machines on the carousel. I hung in there. It came down to a sophomore and me. My freshmen surrounded me, shouting. I won.

Each week it was the same story. They gave me a nickname, sometimes chanting it as the tournament narrowed, "Brutus, Brutus, Brutus!" So, I was hooked.

WRESTLING AND HEART

Dan came the next year and immediately joined the football team. Then I had to talk him into wrestling. He thought the sport was strange. But I persisted, and he joined.

His freshman year Coach Nelson had him wrestle as heavyweight in a particular Junior Varsity tournament. The problem was that on weigh-in day he was too light to make weight. They rejected him at the scales, encouraging us to come back later if we could make it happen. How does a person grow real human tissue in the space of an hour?! Couldn't happen.

So we brought him back to the cafeteria, where, thankfully, he could eat as much as he wanted. Then, when he didn't want anymore, we cheered him on and he downed a few more eggs and pancakes. Just before he got sick, he got up from his chair, stepped on the scale, and made weight. By then he was hungry again, so we all went back to the cafeteria to watch Dan eat some more.

Soon Dan was wrestling on varsity. His junior year he took fourth in the county tournament, which was an accomplishment, considering that San Diego County is bigger than 20 US states.

What happened his senior year was impressive. Dan took first in league and went to the county tournament again. But this time, he was really sick.

The 191-pound finalists in the tournament were monsters. One guy in particular was scary. One whole side of his chest had no hair on it. It was burned off when his radiator blew up on him.

Dan made it to the final match, and won, taking first in the county, but he paid the price. They took him to the hospital in an ambulance. He had won the tournament while suffering from pneumonia. That's heart. He'll talk more about heart later in life.

HIGH SCHOOL

High School became an adventurous routine. Every morning I came over to eat breakfast and ride to school with Dan. His Dad would poach eggs in oil. They were so tasty that way, and when they cooled, you could tuck a whole egg in your mouth. Before long, we took over breakfast duty, each eating a 12-egg omelet with enough cheese and toast to make it work.

As I mentioned, Dan drove long before he was old enough to. His mother died when he was in elementary school, and his dad needed Dan to help him with driving. Dan took on the responsibility, but he was still very young. This made it more fun.

Sometimes when we pulled up to a stop sign I would sing "Stop sign, stop sign!" This was a dare to drive straight through, and Dan never backed away from a dare. Fortunately, the streets of Carlsbad were quiet, and nothing bad ever happened.

The Fa'asamala years were a time of peace at Carlsbad High School. Whenever someone was picked on, they came to Dan, and Dan settled it. The counselors must have loved him. With fights to a minimum, Dan probably spared them reams of suspension and expulsion paperwork, shortening the workday for the entire admin staff by at least 30 minutes. I could imagine Vice Principals and counselors meeting in a local pub after work, toasting young Dan Fa'asamala.

ROGER METZ, THE GURU'S GURU

Naturally, Dan took to the weights. But we both got bored with the cables and levers that were characteristic of high school gyms in those days. And though the school finally acquired some free weights, we were done. We had to find a real gym to train in.

We found Iron Man's Gym on Mission Avenue, downtown Oceanside. The owner was a teacher from Escondido, Roger Metz. Roger was an interesting guy. He had been a Mr. Hawaii in the late 60's—a real bodybuilder! He was also West Coast Editor for Iron Man and one or two other bodybuilding magazines. He also promoted local bodybuilding contests, and, most importantly to Dan's development, arranged seminars of famous bodybuilders.

It might seem a waste that Dan and I landed at a bodybuilding gym rather than a powerlifting gym, but it wasn't about the style. It was about the man. That man was Roger Metz, who became our unofficial guru.

Not only did we learn so much from Roger, but we experienced his sacrifice, his generosity, and his reverent love of human potential. Roger was a rare find in so many ways. He could be critical and demanding, yet positive and hopeful at the same time, like a Steve Jobs of weight lifting.

Iron Man had stacks and stacks of weights. There were benches and squat racks, preacher benches and dumbbells. It also had mirrors on the walls and a lighted stage in the back. By then, we were getting strong, but under the lights, we looked huge. Roger, bodybuilder patrons, and the environment of the gym all got us interested in the sport.

IRON MAN TWINS

We quickly learned that the hardest part about bodybuilding was not the lifting. That was relaxing compared to the real work: dieting. Sure, there were phases when lifting and eating were the bulk of the work, but dieting had to happen sooner or later. In that sport, you not only had to have the muscle, you had to see it.

Wrestling also benefited those who were strong and lean. Since we were cutting weight for wrestling, why not be bodybuilders too?!

Fortunately, we were on the same journey. Without mutual support, we never would have done it. We became known as the Iron Man Twins.

We started training, which meant we started dieting. We learned about the importance of protein. We learned that carbs are evil. We believed that the Atkins diet would help us burn fat and leave muscle.

But we loved frozen yogurt! We started craving coconut frozen yogurt from the shop up the street. So, one day, we threw the whole carb counting thing out the window. We wanted to have a whole day eating coconut yogurt without exceeding our calorie allotment and without shorting our protein needs. So, I got the nutritional information and did the calculation.

The next day Dan and I arrived at the shop when it opened. We left with a large thermos and quarts of Styrofoam cups filled with coconut yogurt. We loved it...for about an hour. Then we got sick of it, but permitted ourselves to eat nothing else all day.

When we started this dieting process, I was a vigorous, enthusiastic 191 lb wrestler. Dan was heavyweight. He started dropping faster than I did. I had to step it up, because I did not want to defend my starting spot against Dan. I dropped one weight class down in time for him to take over 191. Then he was heading for 175, so I dropped a second class to 165. Finally, I was safe at 154 lbs.

Impossible to believe, but Dan was now wrestling at 165, and I was down to 154. I thought I would tear it up at 154—three weight classes down! Instead, I had a miserable 1-5 record, and I felt like a cold wet rag. I had virtually no fat left on me, and yet I probably lost more muscle than fat. I knew I couldn't do both wrestling and bodybuilding, so I quit wrestling. Dan finished the season taking 4th in County, back up to 191 pounds.

The one thing I remember the most from that time was the Natural Teenage America contest. It was in Vegas or Arizona, someplace hot and dry. Dan tied for 5th place, but they needed to resolve it. So they had a pose-down.

This automatically tilted the scale in Dan's favor. Dan loved music, and he always whipped up a fantastic series of poses to go with his songs, poses that featured his strong suits.

The other kid was from New Jersey. The promoters had them pose together. Dan's poses flowed one into the other making the whole show a kind of fluid dance. The other guy got lost in it, fumbling through an awkward routine. He ended up just imitating Dan's poses. But Dan was showing off his huge biceps and his chest, not necessarily the other guy's strengths. Dan won.

FIRST PRINCIPLES

Roger gave Dan and me our first real jobs, as trainers at the gym. We quickly earned his trust and made friends with the gym members. This was fortunate, because Roger included us in every seminar he gave. Roger's pattern was to promote a contest, then, leading up to the contest he would have famous bodybuilders give seminars about their training methods. Most of these guys were former or future Mr. Americas or Mr. Olympias. Often, they would be guest posers at the contests, so they came to present in awesome shape.

We saw Danny Padilla, Sergio Oliva, Serge Nubret, Mike and Ray Mentzer, Kal Szkalak, Tom Platz and more. Even the legendary powerlifter Bill Kazmaier came to the gym. We learned a lot from their seminars. Some of them were blowing smoke. Some told their best secrets. Some claimed they were always steroid free. Others said they did use—had to use—asserting that if anyone said they didn't they were a liar.

One guy said that he had an allergic reaction to steroids, and all he had to do was take the smallest dose, and his body would react by kicking out a whole lot of his own natural testosterone. He turned to his girlfriend who returned his smile. He also claimed his reaction was very dangerous. It could send him into shock, a shock he might never wake out of.

To me, it seemed the most enjoyable and informative seminar was given by Tony Pearson. Tony was genuine. Not only did he give a great talk, but he allowed us all to watch him go through a work-out with his training partner Maury Williams.

Tony and Maury worked purposefully and fast, like longshoremen moving heavy canisters of nuclear fuel. I do not recall any resting between sets, other than when they were shouting encouragements to each other. When one was done, the other jumped on the weight.

Their workout focused on medium-heavy to light weights. There were a lot of sets. It was probably as much a cardio workout as a muscle-building one, comparable to a cross-fit routine, but with more muscles involved — and more sections of muscles involved. Tony believed in attacking a muscle with several lifts, using free weights, cables, whatever would let him hit it from another angle. He and Maury took each set to exhaustion.

When he spoke, Tony spoke honestly. It might have been him who said he trained to build scar tissue. Muscle gets big when you don't give it enough time to heal. The muscle is real muscle, but it's not the same quality as muscle built exclusively for strength.

This was a realization that hit me pretty hard. At that point I decided I was more interested in building strong, efficient, maximally healthy muscle, rather than muscle designed first and foremost to look good on the beach. I think Dan reached that conclusion at the same time. It was about the power.

Tom Platz was also fun to listen to. Of course, what you noticed first about Platz were his legs, giant sweeping thighs. When he posed, not only did the major groups of the thigh separate, but lateral striations popped out all the way along the edges of these muscles. It was crazy! Tom probably influenced the look of all bodybuilders going forward, redefining what "balanced" looked like.

He also showed us how he did it. Squats were important, of course, but what I remember the most was what I call "Platz Squats" He got on a leg machine that had you rest half reclining and half standing up, supporting the weight stack with a padded collar on your shoulders.

As he squatted, HE ROCKED FORWARD ONTO HIS TOES. He kept going down until his knees were far past his feet. Then he reversed direction and rocked back up.

I took that little technique back to my high school gym, where we would occasionally catch a workout. It freaked out my coaches, who thought I would blow out my knees.

I concentrated on my legs as a reaction to my yearbook freshman-wrestling picture. My legs looked so skinny in that picture. I resolved to do something about it. And it worked. At one of Roger's contests I actually took best legs in the division. Thanks Tom!

So, while Tony helped us realize power was more important than size, Tom helped us realize that you can change things that you concentrate on. Moreover, Tom, Tony, and all the rest gave us a much bigger message, and it was exciting: Nothing is set in stone. There is no one right way of doing things. You can find out what works best for you, and maybe, just maybe, you can find out what works best for almost anybody.

DESTROYER OF DESTROYERS

College broke up the Iron Man Twins. I went away to USC while Dan finished his senior year in high school. Our bodybuilding days were done, but we both kept lifting. On summer vacations, I would come home and lift and work with Dan.

Dan got a wrestling scholarship, but turned it down so he could look over his family. He got a job working for a security company. He arranged to get me hired for summers. It was not your typical walk-around-the-parking-lot-at-night kind of a job. In San Diego County there were vast fields of strawberries, flowers, tomatoes and other produce. A certain percentage of the workers on these ranches were migrant workers, some from Mexico, others from Central America. Since the ranches were privately owned, city police would not patrol them. This was unfortunate, because these workers had a propensity for killing each other.

They were mostly nice guys. Most of them lived on the ranches in lean-to's, tents or shacks. They would bring beer in. That put them in the wrong state of mind. Since most of them carried knives, they often settled their arguments with the knives. But the third ingredient that brought things to a head was the putas, the prostitutes. When you throw putas in the mix, it can get deadly.

So, some brilliant entrepreneur got the idea that if they patrolled the ranches, took away the beer, and shooed away the prostitutes, the workers could keep their knives and no one would die. It worked. Sky-high murder rates dropped to zero.

The job was fun and easy, for the most part. Each day the guy who owned the ranch-catering empire lent us his Cadillac. We patrolled the ranches gliding over rutted dirt roads under clear blue California skies.

One day, on one ranch, we approached a campsite. It was the middle of the day, and yet there were two people in a sleeping bag just outside a hut, going at it. That sleeping bag was undulating like a butterfly trying to get out of its cocoon.

We rolled up. I got out and walked toward the bag. When I was a few feet away, they threw down the hood, and I saw two heads looking at me laughing. It was a couple of guys pulling a fast one on us.

Another day we caught a large group of workers red handed—Budweiser red. We crested over a hill just as 8 or 10 of them were carrying cases of beer onto the property. They were Oaxacans. Oaxacans come from a region of Mexico where the people are especially short. From the results of our interaction, I can conclude that Oaxacans are also feisty.

When we got out of the car, I was holding a shotgun. We told the guys we needed the beer. It got silent. Then one of the guys lunged at me, reaching for the gun. I kicked him in the chest. It was on. Dan and the majority of the group were on the other side of the car. I ran to the trunk, threw in the gun, locked it, and raced around to help. As I got there, Dan was on the ground, dealing with someone who tried to hit him. In the meantime, the rest of the group jumped on his back. Dan slowly stood up. The guys started peeling off and sliding down his back. It reminded me clearly of some scene from the Hulk versus the Mole Men—so many of them, yet so small. Who would win? We resolved the scene with only one or two guys being turned over to the police, and we were fine.

That was the hard part of the job. It was physical work, and it led to other jobs. Dan ended up getting bouncer gigs at parties. Invariably, someone had to get thrown out. Occasionally someone would actually challenge Dan to a fight. Oh no, it never worked out for the challenger.

Dan proved to be the real deal. Like Samson, he was not just strong; he knew how to use his strength. Be it the jawbone of an ass or the left hook of an angry bouncer, the result was the same.

Dan was the nicest guy you could ever meet. He was helpful, not easily offended, friendly, and easygoing. But. If you were arrogant; if you were an asshole; things were not likely to go your way.

Sometimes guys who get a drink or two in them think they are invincible. Invincible, they think they are in charge. In charge, they think they can discount anyone. Didn't they see Dan on guard? It never ended up well for them. And Dan enjoyed escorting them out, especially after an incident of humbling.

Dan acquired a reputation of invincibility. People started arranging fights, thinking they would find someone who could beat Dan. Dan continued to despise those who proudly strutted the streets of Oceanside. He took note of the fact that Marines had a reputation of being the baddest bad-asses around. With Camp Pendleton bordering the streets of Oceanside, Dan would often encounter groups of Marines after dark walking around like they owned the place.

He started engaging them. They put forth their toughest, and the toughest went down. Meanwhile, the arranged fights went the same way. Between the Marines, and the other fights, Dan had a record of over 40 matches, never having lost.

This was hard on Dan's girlfriend Karen. Karen eventually married Dan, and gave him his first son, Beau. But in the thick of all this fighting, she was stressed. One weekend, when I was home from school, she asked that we could pray that Dan would stop this fighting.

Soon after, I was driving home from LA. It was midnight on Friday. I knew Dan would be working at 7-11 right off the freeway on Mission Avenue. I decided to pull off and surprise him at work.

He surprised me. As I pulled up, he was standing in the parking lot in front of the 7-11 looking dazed, staring off into the distance. I parked and walked toward him, finally seeing the streams of blood flowing down his face.

Minutes earlier, he had come outside to see what was the fuss between his stepbrother Gnafa and whoever else was outside. When he got outside, a van full of Marines unloaded on Dan. One of them smashed a bottle over his head, giving him a concussion. I imagine a beating ensued, with both parties logging damage. Dan's dad came soon after. He drove Dan to the emergency room at Tri-City Hospital.

3. The Making of a Guru: Mastering

DARKNESS

Dan's last fight was an arranged one. By now, large groups of people would come, one set backing Dan, the other set, the challenger. This last guy was only 175 lbs. — a pushover. But his backers were boisterous and confident. They were excited and ready for a show.

When they started fighting, Dan noticed that the guy's punches stung. He was fast. He landed a lot of jabs. It got loud. The other side was electric, feeling like it was almost over. Their guy had never lost. He was a phenom, and he was doing the same thing he always did.

By now, Dan was getting wobbly. The other guy was hard to hit! He felt himself losing it. He started to fall back. He uppercut with one last haymaker, and landed it. The challenger was out cold.

His people were completely crestfallen, aghast, mouths open, disbelieving. Dan's side was out of control. Raging, they lifted him on their shoulders and carried him out. As Dan looked on the scene, he could feel himself fill with a deep, satisfying pride. Then a thick nauseating darkness descended on him. He knew he had to stop. That was his last fight.

FINDING A PATH

Dan had always been a warrior and a lover. These two aspects of his identity supported one another. He instinctively defended oppressed people from abusers. If there was no one in particular to defend, at least there were bad guys to put down.

But for just an instant, this last fight made him feel like the bad guy. This could not be. At this critical moment, the lover won. Dan snapped back in line with his mission.

Yet Dan never stopped defending, or using physical force to do so. His reputation preceded him. His bouncer work extended to body guarding. He was increasingly called to Las Vegas to guard for various bigwigs on vacation. They paid him $1000 a day for his work: walking around town looking out for his client.

In his personal life, Dan found clearer focus. He committed to God. He cherished his son Beau. He became serious about his work, moving up through the ranks as a guard at the San Onofre Nuclear Power Plant, becoming a supervisor and an alarms expert.

Though his marriage with Karen failed, he eventually married Yvette, taking Yvette's son Sean as his own.

MONSTA GARAGE

Dan never gave up on lifting. He kept lifting in the most convenient place available, his garage. Sometimes his brother Eddie would be with him, and sometimes a couple of other people would show up.

Dan continued to get stronger. Soon, Dan had a regular set of people showing up. He delighted in challenging them. He spotted for each one, keeping track in his mind where each person left off at the previous session. They started to grow too.

More and more people began showing up, predominantly young men from the neighborhood. His own sons Beau and Sean came of age and joined in. Eventually, they reached the limit for one bar. It took too long to rotate 15 or 20 guys through the routine, so Dan got another bench.

He designated one of his strong men to be spotter over the second bench. The second bench handled the newcomers. Once the lifter could rep with a plate on each side, he was welcome to step up to the big bar. It became a kind of initiation ceremony, a happy event for the ascender.

Remembering where each lifter was in his development was a huge task — especially for someone who didn't believe in writing things down. Like an underground bookie, Dan had a knack for keeping things in his mind. But a lot more was going on in his head.

Dan was doing scientific experiments on his men. Consciously or not, he tweaked the workouts, honing each variable until it optimized the gains. He went from three days a week to two days. He observed the results of various grip widths and thumb positions, set numbers, and rest periods.

What made a difference on injuries, strength gains, and motivation — all these caught his attention. But again, nothing was written down. He kept it all in his head, with supporting evidence piling up in the muscle growing around him in Monsta Garage.

WE DON'T TRAIN BULLIES. WE EAT BULLIES.

Some days, Dan would also teach interested lifters how to box, and just how to fight. Some stayed around for these lessons, or came back the next day to spar.

With this group of guys getting strong and skilled, they acquired that summonable power that Dan always held in high regard. But he also understood it could be misused, and he would have none of that. This is what he told me about his Monster Making philosophy:

> It's all about representing not only this garage, but...when you start working with 300 lbs, or 200 lbs actually, you become dangerous. There are expectations I have. I definitely don't want to hear that you are a bully.
>
> We don't train bullies. We eat bullies. I definitely don't want to hear that you are a bully or anything like that. I check how you talk or how you are when you are with us. And I definitely will maintain that. There's no way I'm going to train a monster to go out there and be like that, or you won't be allowed to lift here. You can do that anywhere else, but you won't do that here.

The guys who stuck around were either attracted to that sentiment, or grew into it. Either way, it was good.

CHAMPIONS

Eventually, some of the lifters started achieving world-class power. From 1999 through 2003 four Monstas from Dan's garage took 5 world records at the Amateur Athletic Union's bench press competitions. This information is summed up in a table at the end of the chapter. When a world record was made, the table implies an American record as well.

Furthermore, the Monsta lifters compete exclusively in the "Raw" category, which just means the lifters wear no assistive clothing. Years ago some lifters started wearing springy Kevlar vests during competitions. These made such a difference that AAU introduced a new category they called "Equipped". Usually, Monsta raw records were big enough to take the equipped category too, but I make no mention of these records in the table. Furthermore, lifters in AAU competition had to submit to drug testing to guarantee that the lift was achieved by natural training methods.

The first Monsta with a United States record was Jason Padgette. Competing in the 16-17 age group and the 181 lb. weight class, Jason got the record with a 341-pound bench. Jason currently weighs in the mid-200's. At 32 years of age, he could make a run at another record. I have seen him rep in the 500s.

Next up, Beau, Dan and Karen's son, established a world record in the 14-15 age group. At 275 pounds, he pressed 380.3 pounds. Soon after, Beau got the 16-17 year old, 275-pound weight class world record, set at 402.34 pounds.

Dan himself represented Monsta with his world record lift in the Masters 40-44 year old, 308+ lb weight class. He pressed 550.99 pounds. Since then Dan has lifted over 620 pounds in the garage. Unfortunately, a catastrophic injury will most likely prevent Dan from ever putting that weight up in an official venue. Still, the Monstas know their Guru has come within a hundred pounds of the unlimited, un-drug-tested all-time all-world record of approximately 720 pounds.

Sean, Dan's other son, achieved a world record that Dan believes will be held for a long, long time. At only 181 pounds, and competing in the 20-23 year old age group, Sean pressed 418 pounds. When he set that record, the officials immediately whisked Sean away for drug testing. Dan said, "Go ahead, you aren't gonna find anything in that kid but a whole bunch of Big Macs."

Jason Padgette set the next Monsta world record. Now in the 18-19 year old category, and slightly heavier at 198 pounds, Jason put up 363.7 pounds.

THE PRESENT

At this writing I have been driving up to Monsta now for a little over a year. I have taken some formal interviews with various Monstas. I have asked some casual questions, and I've participated in a lot of frivolous banter. So I feel that I have both my history right and a true feel for what Monsta Gym is about.

I am now bringing four others with me from San Diego: two friends from work, Joe and Adrian, and my own sons, Alex and Jonathan. Alex is 23 years old, 6 foot, 4 inches tall, with a very lean build. Dan dubbed him "The Phenom" for two reasons: 1) He came from nowhere to knock, of all people, me, his father. Beating me two workouts in a row, he put up 285 lbs. 2) People see him lift and find it hard to believe that a guy so lanky can move so much weight. He won't look that way for long. Once guys at Monsta start repping 285 lbs, they get thick.

Jonathan just started but is making gains. Joe, helping a friend, got hit with a jackhammer injury early on, but he's already past where he started. Adrian is repping well over 200 lbs.

And there is talk of a fresh run at records. Jordan is getting close to record weight with a body weight of 140 lbs. Jarrad, a light-hearted competitor with Alex, is accelerating as fast or faster than anyone there. In just a handful of months, I have seen him go from not being able to do a rep with two plates, to clearing 285 lbs.

The Monday and Friday lifts are getting big again, with as many as 18 guys showing up. It might be time to drag the second bench out of mothballs.

THE RECORDS

All records are raw, with no assistive gear:

Jason Padgette, 1999, American Record, ages 16-17, 181 lbs., **341 lbs. bench**
Beau Fa'asamala, 2000, World Record, ages 14-15, 275 lbs., **380.3 lbs. bench**
Beau Fa'asamala, 2000, World Record, ages 16-17, 275 lbs., **402.33 lbs. bench**
Dan Fa'asamala, 2000, World Record, ages 40-44, 308+ lbs., **550.99 lbs. bench**
Sean Fa'asamala, 2002, World Record, ages 20-23, 181 lbs., **418 lbs. bench**
Jason Padgette, 2003, World Record, ages 18-19, 198 lbs., **363.7 lbs. bench**

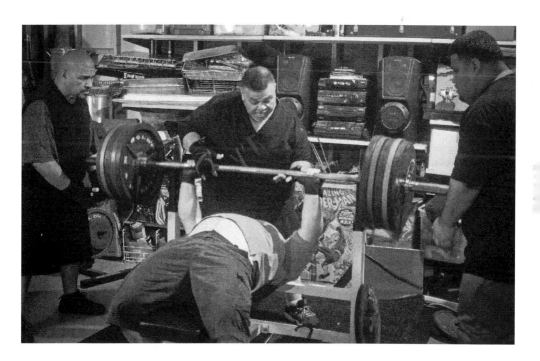

Part II: GURU'S PRACTICE

4. Technique

POWER: THE GOAL

Doubtless, there are some people who might strip everything away from this book, leaving only this one chapter. Indeed, this chapter is the how-to guide to achieve, mechanically, physically, the amazing muscle growth of Monsta Garage. But to look only here would be a mistake. Each of us is more than a flesh and blood analog of a machine. Humans need more than a simple set of operating instructions. The following chapters on *motivation*, *coaching*, and *heart* are essential to reaching the highest degree of performance.

Yet when it comes to building power, this *is* how Monsta does it. Before I describe each technique in detail I need to make a clear distinction between goals: One obvious lifter's goal is power, another is breaking records. Paradoxically, the two goals are not exactly the same.

To open the book, I presented Dan and Monsta's first foray into AAU competition. AAU's Martin Drake had much praise for Dan and the gym. However, he did have some critique. Martin asserted that Dan and his guys could each add 50 to 60 pounds to their lifts, if they just paid attention to a couple of points relevant to the competition. So, as a bonus to those interested in pursuing records, as well and to distinguish between the two goals, here I present Martin's suggestions. Each is totally legal for competition, and each is widely practiced, except by the Monsta men—for reasons outlined below.

First, Dan's men could lift more if they rocked and inflated their upper torsos, thereby decreasing the distance from bar to chest. The physics is obvious: Energy is force times distance. Less distance means less work is required to complete the lift.

Second, The Monstas could hoist a bigger load if they didn't wait so long to press from the chest to full extension. AUU judges require the lowered bar to become still before they give the command to press. This normally takes a second or a second and a half. Dan's men wait from four to five seconds before pushing.

I asked Dan why he doesn't take advantage of what the competition allows. He says it is intentional, and it is about the goal: Power. He practices a purity of form that reflects this message even during competition. If a full range press brings the lifter full development of power, why should he alter form for competition?

Ironically, Dan learned by competing that the pause before pressing did in fact demonstrate raw power. That is when he became an avid advocate of the pause. While the pause is not necessary for training, Dan does believe it is necessary to demonstrate true power—he just takes it to the extreme by insisting on a couple of extra seconds of stillness preceding each competition lift.

Once again, to Dan and the Monstas, it's about the power, not the record. Nevertheless, the records do come. What follows are the techniques that build power, the kind of power that breaks records regardless.

CLOSE GRIP WITH SUICIDE GRIP

Imagine you are in a machine shop. You turn to see a large steel tool chest towering to a height of 7 feet. Some prankster pushes it from behind and it starts to fall on you. It's too late to get out of the way. What do you do? You reach up and stop it. In your mind's eye, where do you see your hands? How are they positioned? I would bet that you instinctively put your hands up in the same way you would lift weights in Monsta Garage. You do this even if you've never lifted in Monsta Garage! This is the close-grip with suicide grip hand position (CGSG).

It's the same way offensive linemen push during a pass rush. It's the same way a sumo wrestler pushes, unless he's tangled up with the arms of the other wrestler.

Under none of these situations do people put their elbows out to the side or make their forearms 90 degrees from their upper arms, as in the standard bench press. Nor do these natural situations require the thumb to stretch in a grasping or clutching position. Instead, whether pushing a tool chest, a lineman or a sumo wrestler, the thumb is likely to be resting comfortably near the rest of the fingers.

Why is this hand position superior? Because it generates the most power. A traditional wide grip bench press isolates the pectorals more than the CGSG does. This might seem paradoxical to the reader, since I am using world bench-press records as evidence that the methods of Monsta Gym produce the most power. But not really. If my claim is that the CGSG is better than the traditional bench at developing power, and if Monsta trains primarily with the CGSG over the traditional bench, and yet superior results are achieved on the traditional bench, this speaks volumes about the supremacy of the CGSG.

As a musician and a bass player, I recognize the best guitarists, bassists, and even drummers often have a background in piano. Piano training is an awesome developer of music theory, musical ear, and rhythm. Similarly, CGSG is an optimal developer of upper body power. The traditional bench press is one measure of this power.

The first time I had 285 lbs on the bar at Monsta Gym, I noticed that the CGSG absolutely mashed my frontal deltoids at the bottom of the lift. I also noticed in the months to follow that my shoulders, triceps, and chest all gained size from this lift. The CGSG trades emphasis on each of these muscle groups throughout the rep. This is not nearly so true with the traditional wide grip. See the discussion on "the line" at the end of this section for more on this.

Here is how CGSG is done. First the close-grip part: The traditional close grip is designed for concentration of force on the triceps, for the development of the back of the arm. Dan has his people hold the bar further out than the traditional close-grip, maybe even closer to traditional "wide-grip" bench press hand position. Hands hold the bar slightly further than shoulder width. Here's what Dan says about it:

> Close grip back in the day for us was really so close that it put so much unnecessary pressure on your elbows. That kind of workout was mainly for bodybuilders. But we are trying to build power.

Second comes the "suicide" part of the CGSG, so called because the thumb is kept on the same side of the bar as the rest of the hand. To some, it might seem that an untimely sneeze in the middle of the lift could set the bar to sliding down the lifter's forearms leading to a catastrophic landing, possibly on the lifter's face. Not that that couldn't happen, but I defer that discussion to the "Safe is Sexy" section of Chapter 6.

Dan compares the suicide grip to the ergonomics of the curl bar. He says the suicide grip resolves unnecessary tensions, concentrating the force where it belongs. Injuries subside with the close grip. And, fewer injuries mean more consistency in training, which translates to bigger gains. Here is what Jason says about the suicide grip and the CGSG in general:

Burtson:
> Do you feel it is effective?

Padgette:

> Absolutely. Just like I can feel the difference between when I do that and when I wrap the fingers around — just like I can feel the difference when I do wide grip and close grip. We used to do only five to seven sets of close grip (with suicide grip) and eight to twelve sets of wide grip.

> We were getting a number or shoulder injuries. So we do the opposite now, more close grip and less wide grip. Now we haven't had those issues with our shoulders.

Here I will make a very subtle and previously overlooked point about how to make the CGSG approximate the most natural, safest, power-accessing push: eliminate the straight bar itself. This might be the last frontier in benching power. Dan mentioned the ergonomics of the curl bar. Why not apply that to the bench bar? If you look at natural hand placement, optimal positioning would likely allow for a slight angling outward of the two hands. There are two pieces of evidence to support this claim:

1) Martial arts teach you to punch so that the knuckles of your index and middle fingers are in alignment with the two bones of the lower arm. Why? — for safety, to provide a foundation for the expression of maximum power, and to create a more fluid punch. Note that if you hold both hands together in proper punch position, a straight bar could not go through them.

2) I have often seen the best lifters at Monsta rotate the hands slightly outward during the close grip with suicide grip. This is possible because the grip allows the base of the hand to provide the main support for the bar, freeing the fingers to loosen and rotate, en-masse, outward.

The effectiveness of the CGSG push makes even more sense in context of what Dan calls *the line*. A few months ago, I did a clean rep with 285 lbs. Dan had me do it again on my next set. I had never done a third set in series with this weight, but he had me try it again. This time, he made me aware of the line, and coached me through it, so that I got the rep for a third time.

The line is a technique that not only enables a person to lift more than he normally would, but it is part of the package of developing the person to the fullest.

The line is actually a plane, for you geometry buffs. It represents the path taken by the bar on the way up from the chest to rep completion. It starts with the bar positioned about a half inch to an inch below the nipple line and proceeds up in a straight line at a slight angle towards the head.

We already dealt with why the close-grip/suicide-grip is ideal for development: it utilizes three major upper body muscle groups: the pectorals (upper and lower), the triceps, and the frontal deltoids. Now, with attention to the line, these three muscle groups get the proper respect. At different times through the rep, one set of muscle is dominant in the power it provides. Others are helpers. But throughout that one rep, other sets of muscles become dominant, leaving the former dominant ones just minor players. This not only puts peak stress on all the muscles, but it allows them each in turn to share less in the duration of that stress. It's like running. What's going to give you bigger leg development, doing a sprint or a marathon? The sprint puts big stress on the muscles and exhausts them quickly.

Dan also encourages the lifter to get the bar moving fast along the line. My guess on the reason for this is that the established momentum takes the bar through those iffy transition zones where one major group relinquishes power as the next group takes over the load.

So each group in turn gives all it has, maximizing overall available power. To every force there is an equal and opposite force. This means that as each muscle maximally contributes to the lift, it also gets worked to its utmost—a win-win for present and future power.

So it is with the line. If you are going to push with a certain grip, you have to understand that the path of the push is specific to that push. The line simply follows the path along which the muscles most efficiently trade the lead during a CGSG push.

Close Grip With Suicide Grip, Summarized:

- Grip the bar slightly wider than shoulder width.
- Keep the thumbs on the same side of the bar as the rest of the fingers.
- Do not try to spread elbows outward. Let them be where they naturally separate.
- Let the bar touch the chest at from one-half to one inch below the nipple line.
- Push up in a straight line angled slightly towards the head.

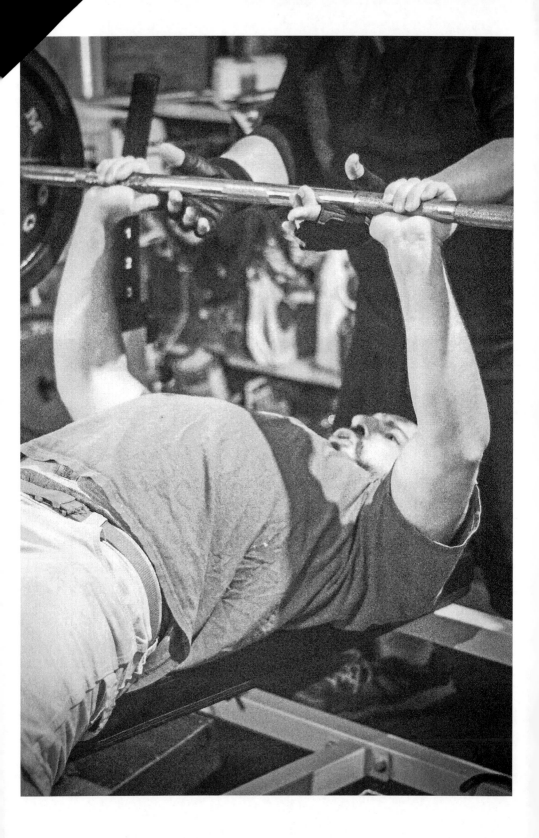

THE LADDER

Occasionally, Monsta Gym will get visitors who are already very strong. They've heard about the gym and stop by for various reasons. Maybe they've hit a plateau and want to see how they can get higher.

This happened recently. A man named Steve dropped by for his first lift at Monsta. He had huge, sweeping, hypertrophied muscle, looking like someone drawn by a comic book artist. That night he was repping a few plates—eventually.

But first, he had to go through the same low weight warm ups that are a part of the Monsta ladder. No matter who you are or how much you can lift, you've got to start with just the bar and only a 45-pound plate on each end. Then you've got to stay there for two sets. Next, you have to do two more sets with only that and a 25 on each side. This is where beginners peak, but the 500+ lifters go to sets 5 and 6 with "only" two plates on each side.

More people stay at that weight, but others go on to 2 plates and a quarter. After repping three plates, then they might jump to 5 plates if they want to go that heavy.

Everyone peaks, staying 2-3 sets at a weight they can do 2-5 times, then the weights get lower.

By the end of the night, each lifter will have done 12-14 sets. I asked Dan why he started so low. He said,

> Warm up and respect for the weight. . . I do a four minute call for warm up, but . . . not everybody's warming up or stretching. So, in essence, it's just a good and safe way to get them to stretch and get warmed up. We start off with the bar (bar plus 45s on each side), which is ridiculous, because my top four guys probably don't even feel the bar.

Dan acknowledges that is extraordinary, as it seemed foreign to Steve that night. Several times, on the slow rise up the ladder, Steve asked if higher weights could be placed on the bar. Dan said something like, "soon, you'll be up repping 700 lbs, but for now. . ." Steve did the low weights.

Currently, Jason is Monsta's strongest lifter. When I was talking to him about squats, he said that he used to do them, but one day he came up too quickly and tore his thigh. At first I thought he meant he thrust up from squat position too fast. He actually meant that he hadn't gone slowly up the ladder Monsta-style, and he paid the price.

The ladder is not a new invention, but the Guru of Monsta garage insists on it, despite complaints that it starts too low, and other complaints that it steals strength from the higher lifts. The ladder also helps maintain the health of the ligaments and tendons. See more about the importance of having strong, healthy ligaments and tendons in Chapter 6.

Monsta's ladder probably does start lower than most strong lifters are used to, but maybe it also keeps more lifters injury free. Uninterrupted, they go on to make bigger and bigger gains.

The Ladder, Summarized:

- Lifting starts with a 4-minute call for stretching.
- All lifters start with just the bar and a plate on each side.
- Weights go up in 50 or 90 pound increments until each lifter is at his peak range, repping 2-5 times.
- The other side of the ladder has lifters coming back down in weight, doing more reps again.
- The down side of the ladder has fewer sets than the up side.
- 12-14 sets comprise the workout, from warm up to warm down.

VARIABILITY IN REST BETWEEN SETS

A lot of people confuse consistency and variability. They think that to lock down gains they have to be scientific, use writing pads and stop watches, and wear a lab coat. They insist on order, regularity. Keeping all conditions constant, they look for one more rep with the same weight, or maybe one more five-pound plate with the same number of reps. I know these people exist, because I used to be one, and it only got me so far.

Sure, what happens to your body is science. But what happens in the gym needs to look more like a stormy sea than a lab room. When Dan turns on that boom box, sometimes I think I can hear Thor pounding his hammer, making thunder and lightning. Don't worry about what's happening at the cellular level. Be in the gym. Stress your body.

There is a bigger science in the disorder, in the messiness of the gym environment. Regardless of who shows up, regardless of how many people come to lift, the Power Guru would recommend that you go with the flow. If you wait exactly 90 seconds between sets, the body gets used to that. The body needs to be tricked into growing. You have to surprise it, stress it in a way that breaks a pattern. The body is efficient. It will use muscle as fuel. It will burn that muscle unless it thinks it needs it to deal with the next unpredictable trauma you put it through. Regular timing between sets is one of those patterns that needs to be broken up. Jason agrees:

> As far as the sets and reps and jumps, I think the most important thing is to not stick to one particular thing...You've got to change up your workouts.

And that changing up happens naturally from work out to work out depending on how many people show up. Sometimes there have been only two people. I've been there with 18. Six or seven seems ideal, but ranging from 2 to 18 is better than a regular group of six or seven.

With only two people lifting you might have less than a minute of rest between sets. With 18, you might be waiting for ten minutes. The result is that one day you are exhausting your muscles quickly. The next you give the muscles time to recharge, and you can keep the weights higher. This is a shock, and it's good.

Variability In Rest Between Sets, Summarized:

- Lifters move quickly on and off the bench to keep the rest times manageably short.
- Lifters tolerate randomly varying rest periods, established by how many people show up.
- When 20 or more people start showing up on a regular basis, it's time to get a second bench.

VARIABILITY IN NUMBERS OF REPS IN A SET

Number of reps is another variable that benefits power via random shocks. Dan programs the variation two ways. The first way is conventional. More reps are done on the warm ups and the fewest happen at the peak weight. The lightest warm ups should go for at least ten reps a set. Intermediate weights might require six to ten reps. These go to failure. That last rep is a struggle. Dan likes to shoot for from 2 to 5 reps at the peak weight.

The second way the Power Guru programs random rep counts is by making spontaneous declarations of special lifts. There are three of these: *follow the leader*, the *pause-rep* and big weight repping.

Approximately once every three lifting sessions Dan will call for *follow the leader* sets. It's always at the end of the workout taking up the last two or three sets. He, or someone high in the hierarchy will do as many reps as he can with some mid-to light weight. For example, with 235 lbs on the bar one of the stronger lifters might get 25 reps. The challenge is for the next two lifters to get the same 25. If one of these guys gets only 24, Dan calls out "Zero"!

To make it fair, Dan might lower the weight by 50 or 90 pounds for the next few lifters in the hierarchy. A different change-up would be to make the next three guys total 25 reps with the 235-pound weight. The people at the end of the line might shoot for 25 reps with the bar and the 25s. You are allowed to cheat by using short strokes on *follow the leader* as long as it's not blatant. Too many zeros and the workout goes on longer.

The *pause-rep* is more rare than *follow the leader*. When it's called, it also takes place towards the end of the workout. Here, lifters bring a medium heavy weight down holding it (not resting it) on his chest. Dan watches the bar go still. In three or four seconds he gives a shout letting the lifter push the weight up. One to five reps are called out until the lifter can do no more. This is difficult, and often results in a special soreness the next day.

Occasionally the Guru will help the lifter do a lot of reps with his peak weight. That means that by the end of the set, the Guru will be lifting a lot of the weight himself. "Occasionally" and "a lot" will be left for your interpretation and adaptation.

Variability In Numbers Of Reps In A Set, Summarized:

- Lifters vary rep counts through the workout, starting with at least ten reps on the lightest warm-up weights.
- Lifters press intermediately heavy weights to exhaustion, going for six to ten reps.
- The Guru challenges lifters with a peak weight chosen to bring about exhaustion between two and five reps into the set.
- Similar rep counts apply to going back down the ladder.
- The Guru calls for *follow-the-leader* sets once every three or so workouts.
- The Guru calls for *pause-rep* sets once a month or so.
- Occasionally the Guru will help the lifter do a lot of reps with his peak weight.

CONCENTRATION ON ONE LIFT

When I came to Monsta Garage, it was with a humble attitude. Who could criticize anything about a gym with such dramatic results? I reminded myself of this by acknowledging it as the best gym on the planet.

But the one thing that seemed peculiar to me was the insistence on doing just *one lift*. This was hard for me for a number of reasons. One, we used to be bodybuilders! One of the goals of a body builder is to build the body—the whole body!

As much as I respected our guru Roger Metz, I remember once clearly defying him. I saw a picture of a bodybuilder on the cover of a magazine and I said, "What's that?" I was looking at a little muscle on the outer part of the upper arm called the *brachialis*. It sits between the biceps and the triceps. I thought, "I need to develop that!"

I read up on the brachialis and learned that reverse grip curls would do the trick. Roger was a minimalist himself, believing in a few basic power building lifts. He saw me doing the reverse curls and strongly discouraged me. Dan and I were just finishing our workout anyway. We were putting away the weights, but I couldn't let it go. As Roger walked into the back, I started doing reverse curls with the 45-pound plate I happened to have in my hands! For the next year or two I continued to over train, naively believing that more was better. Soon however, Dan and I got wiser and started to simplify, even at this young age.

Another reason one lift didn't make sense was because I understood Dan highly esteemed power, especially functional power, say, the kind you needed when you had to lift a car off someone, or when you needed to throw somebody out of a club.

I wondered about just doing the bench press. Is that going to give you a big chest and nothing else? Fighters depend on back strength as much as chest strength. So how does a person justify one lift?

After being there a year, I now understand how it works. But I asked a lot of questions about this in my interviews. I got my answers.

During this part of my first interview with Dan I was talking specifically about the close-grip with suicide-grip, why it works.

Burtson:
>I was thinking about where I am sore; where I feel the pressure when I lift this way. I feel it on my front delts, triceps, and chest. . .

Fa'asamala:
>What I like about that is you do get a workout on your chest; you are still getting good coverage and foundation—back-up for the rest of your body. That's what's great about our workout. And that's why people—I think you've noticed—their builds are so thick from the side. . .And just that technique hits the body better, and your body actually supports that lift better because of the way it's set up. That's what I've seen over the years.

Burtson:
>Will other lifts help, hurt, or not matter?

Fa'asamala:
> I've had other people do those things, like Jay, my number-one guy. And like anything else, it will take away, power-wise. It will take a little bit away. But it all depends on what you want. We're considered specialists because we focus and concentrate on the bench. But the way we work out contributes to the rest of the body—your abs, your upper body.

Burtson:
> I feel it in my lats even.

Fa'asamala:
> Everything we do, because we do so many reps and sets. If you think about it that way, you are actually working your whole body. Remember *Three sets and you're done*? Three sets and we're not even warmed up.

Alex Burtson:
> Does this work the same muscles as when you do pull-ups?

Fa'asamala:
> Not in the same way, but you are hitting those same muscles in a different direction.

Burtson:
> I know, I look at Jay and how thick he is and Peter, I know they are getting some stimulation.

Fa'asamala:
> Those guys don't do anything else but this. Think about it.
> Look at Jay; he's a monster! This is all he does. That's what I'm talking about. That's how funny this is!
>
> Jay entered a bodybuilding competition, and I have his trophy here. He took 3rd place. He didn't have any legs, or he would have been first. We don't work legs. We used to back in the day.
>
> But that's my point. You look at these guys. Wait till you see big John, he's just another big mass, like me, we're just thick that way. John doesn't do anything else. He can sit here and do 20 reps with 400 lbs. But because of his inconsistency, it takes him a while to start up. But my point is, yeah, look at these guys.

That's why I wanted you too look at Pete, mainly Pete, because Pete was as skinny if not skinnier than you (Alex). But he stayed with this system, and look at him now.

And he'll even tell you, *Oh, I'm not as big as I used to be.* He's right! Most people will look at him thinking, *This is a skinny guy? . . .that's a pretty thick skinny guy! . .* .Well, you look at Pete. Pete's pretty thick and he's 6-4, 6-5? . . . He's a formidable individual, and it's a good thing he's got a good heart. . .

There is no question Pete is thick. See the description of teak wood arms in Chapter One. What I appreciate most about this interview is the recollection of the time Jay (Jason) competed in a bodybuilding contest and came in third. His photo revealed a balanced, bulging physique. His legs weren't small, but not in contest shape. He really might have won had he added squats as a second lift!

I asked Jason, AAU bench press world record holder, why he entered that one bodybuilding contest. Jason replied:

> One of my friends talked me into it. At that time I was about 280, 290 pounds. I really wanted to lose that body weight and see where I was . . .It took a year to cut down to 205.

He learned that "where (he) was," was an overall strong, balanced physique. Later in life, Jason did try other lifts. I asked him about this.

Burtson:
    What other method of lifting appeals to you?

Padgette:
    Powerlifting. I used to do squats and deadlifts as well. The big three. I did those mainly back in 2005.

Burtson:
    Did it compete with your upper body or did it enhance it?

Padgette:
    It's hard to say. I know I put the most weight on when I started incorporating squats and deadlift. My bodyweight jumped up about 20 pounds within six months or so. I was literally putting about 25 pounds on my lifts every week for a while there.

Burtson:
    Did that impact your bench as well?

Padgette:
> My bench was going up, but not as fast.

Note that Jason got his world record years before he experimented with the full set of three power lifts.

There is one technical detail that needs to be clarified: Dan's Monstas actually do two versions of the bench press. The bread and butter piece is the close-grip with suicide-grip bench. The other lift is the standard wide-grip bench press.

They used to do more standard bench than close-grip (See Jason's quote.) Now, the garage only does two sets every other workout—after they've come down the ladder doing close-grip. However, over the last few months, they've tossed even that out the window. It's all about the close-grip with suicide-grip bench press for power.

Concentration on one lift, summarized:

- Do only the CSGS.
- Throw in a couple of sets of standard bench towards the end of the workout, once a week.
- If you are competing in bench press competitions, increase the proportion of sets that are standard bench, as the competition approaches.

CONSTANT TENSION

Constant tension is another aspect of lifting at Monsta Garage that you likely wouldn't see anywhere else. It's a simple technique. Instead of lifting until arms are straight, the lifter never locks the elbows. People who are new to the garage have a hard time with this, so the lead spotter (Dan) will hold an open hand at the proper height for the lifter. After lifting to the hand for a few sets, the lifter usually gets the proper feel. If you are trying this in your own gym, shoot for your forearm to be about 30 degrees from full extension.

Constant tension goes all the way back to our time at Iron Man's gym. It was then that Roger, our mentor, adopted a lifting style that sought to maximize intensity over a very short time span. He got it from Harold Poole, a former training partner and an IFBB Mr. Universe and Mr. America back in the early '60s.

Here's how Roger would do his maximum intensity workout.

First, he'd start with a good general warm up. Then he would do one set, *one set*, for each major body part.

Roger had a number of injuries from his college gymnastic days, so he always took time to wrap his elbows. He could not depend on a spotter, since he had such a busy life teaching and running the gym. He liked doing bench on a machine that had him sit upright. He put on a heavy weight. Then, he would explode on the set and work it until he could do no more. The set was intense all the way through. He maintained that intensity by not relieving the stress at the end of each rep. His arms stayed slightly bent with the motion gently reversing like a ball thrown into the air, reaching its peak and turning around.

It is hard to say how important constant tension is. You can feel how hard the CGSG hits your major upper body muscles. That's a no-brainer, but does maintaining stress throughout a set give the lifter a developmental advantage? You'll have to take the word of Poole, Metz, and Fa'asamala, quite a lineage.

However, if you take the concept of maximum intensity and look for it in everything Monsta does, you'll see it everywhere: Peaking at heavy weights, assisted repping at the peak, concentration on one lift, and the CSGS. It's also in variable rests between sets, and of course, it's in constant tension.

Perhaps one reason Monsta Gym commits to one lift is the implicit understanding that a human only has so much intensity to give. Therefore intensity is invested in the one exercise that promises the maximum potential in human power. Constant tension is another way to concentrate that intensity on the bench.

Constant Tension, Summarized:

- Do not let your arms extend completely at the top of a rep.
- Let gravity reverse your motion when your arms are about 30-degrees short of extension.
- Have the lead spotter use his hand as a target for the inexperienced lifter.

CONSISTENCY

There weren't too many Monsta-like humans walking around my college campus back in the 80's. But I did notice one. He looked like he stepped off the stage at the Olympia, threw on slacks and a button-down shirt, and got teleported to the plaza at UCSD. I saw this guy a few times, but never ran into him in the gym.

Unfortunately for me, trying to lift at that college was like taking a step back in time. I was back to machines, no free weights. That's probably why I never ran into that guy in the gym. I'm sure he found a real gym to work out in; otherwise I would have asked how he got so big.

But one day, a few years later, I was at a wedding with my buddy Tom Graham. Tom is one of the naturally strongest people I have ever met. He can squat seismically active stacks of steel. His dad was a famous villain pro wrestler back in the 50s and 60s, "Dr. Jerry Graham." He wore sequin-covered capes and hypnotized his opponents before throwing them over the ropes.

Tom and I both noticed this guy at another table. You couldn't miss him. He looked like a suit stuffed with bricks. Even his face was angular, like he had a robotic metal faceplate under his flesh. We got up and surrounded him at the reception.

After catching up on our common alma mater, we asked him a series of questions. He had two subtle straight, symmetrical scars on each cheek. We asked him about those. In an English accent he explained he was born in a village in Nigeria. When a young man approaches adulthood, he has the option to be declared a warrior. He goes through a ritual, and he has to kill a lion. He has to hunt the lion down, and kill him with a spear. If you are successful, you become a warrior, and you get those scars on your face.

How bad-ass is that!? We were mesmerized.

Eventually we asked him "How do you do it? How do you stay so huge?!" He said, "I have one word, 'consistency'."

It is that important. That's why *consistency* ends this chapter on technique. Without it, nothing gets done. Jason Padgette agrees with the lion killer.

Burtson:
>You guys do a certain number or sets, reps, jumps, hierarchy, lifts you do and do not do, spotter techniques, two days a week — which of these is the most effective? Even how you grip the bar . . .

Padgette:
>Consistency.

The Power Guru says something similar. He says it this way:

I used to have these guys working out hard. I had them sweating, and I let them know, when their heads were down. *Think about it, your competition, no matter what you compete in, I promise you, pretty much right now, they are sitting in front of the TV with a Twinkie, while you are sitting here working out.*

That's what you've got to say to yourself, "There's no way I can lose! I'm putting in the effort, the work, going out of my way to do what I gotta do."

So, that should drive you to be that much more successful. Your putting in the work, putting in the time, just gives you that little bit of an edge. Think about it. My competition, no matter what it is we end up competing in, there's no way he's working out as hard as me. There's no way he's committing as much as I am.

Though the Monsta gym crowd favors power, that doesn't take anything away from the bodybuilders. They made an impression on me from the seminar days. They are committed. Even so, most of them said breaks are necessary. The standard prescription was to take a one or two week break from lifting once or twice a year. Still, that's a far cry from a two-week break once a month.

Take it from Woody Allen: "Eighty percent of success is showing up." You could come to the best gym on the planet 26 times a year, and you could be beat by the guy who consistently does his pushups twice a week. Show up.

But for Monsta gym I have to add a second layer of consistency. There's lifting weights hard twice a week. That's level one. Then there's lifting weights hard at Monsta gym twice a week, that's level two.

Monsta has something special about it. This will be clear in later chapters. You try harder; you lift more at Monsta. When I can't make it to Oceanside, I will catch a lift, but it always seems I can't do as much weight or as many reps as when I am at Monsta gym. This book would not exist if there weren't something special about the process and the aura you find at Monsta.

Consistency is one of the few concepts in this book that can be generalized to bring about mastery in all aspects of your life. Listen to Danny: "My competition, no matter what it is we end up competing in . . . there's no way he's committing as much as I am."

I highly recommend a book that's really about this one issue, consistency: *The War of Art*, by Steven Pressfield. I close this section with a quote from the book: "It's better to be in the arena, getting stomped by the bull, than to be up in the stands or out in the parking lot." Or at home with a Twinkie.

Consistency, Summarized:

- Lift twice a week, no less, every week.
- Whenever possible, make your lifting happen in a place where you are acknowledged, and where people care about each other's progress.
- Take one or two weeks off once or twice a year, no more.

5. Motivation and Consistency

If you are reading this book because you want to get strong, and if you really, really, really want that physical power, you might as well skip this section, because you will find a way to make it happen. However, if you are a coach, a trainer, a parent, a lifting partner, or you want to be a power guru yourself, you might pick up a few tips on how to motivate people. No matter who you are, definitely check out the *Hierarchy* and *Camaraderie* sections.

This chapter is really an answer to the last section of the last chapter: *Consistency*. Consistency is of utmost importance. Again, I'm plugging the Pressfield book when I say that you have to treat the pursuit of a goal like war. When the generals call for action, they mean it. The troops have to be ready and they have to make it happen. Every time. But the generals are not the ones who are going to storm the hill. The soldiers are. The soldiers have to go from sleeping in their skivvies to running with their assault rifles in seconds, if need be. They are trained to make that happen. They are put through hell. They are drilled. They cannot decide to take the day off. When they are called, they go. Your lifters are the soldiers. And their battle, their war, is a personal one, for them and for them alone. Without motivation they will have no consistency. Without consistency they will lose.

Here's one adaptation of a quote from General Patton in his "Speech to the Third Army":

> Now there's another thing I want you to remember. I don't want to get any messages saying that *we are holding our position*. We're not holding anything. Let the Hun do that. We are advancing constantly and we're not interested in holding onto anything except the enemy. We're going to hold onto him by the nose and we're going to kick him in the ass. We're going to kick the hell out of him all the time and we're going to go through him like crap through a goose!

That's motivational. That's making it happen. I want to be on that team. If you want power, you are going to lift, no question.

But how do we get lifters to lift consistently? We can't train them like soldiers. There are federal laws against going absent without leave, but not for skipping a workout. Since we can't make it illegal for them to skip, we have to motivate them.

TWO KINDS OF MOTIVATION

I have spent 20 years in the world of education. My biggest assignment has been teaching physics. Physics used to be a class taken by a few seniors, but where I teach it became mandatory for freshmen. You could imagine the motivation problems with freshmen in physics.

To deal with the challenge, I directed my Master's thesis on exactly that issue with "Pull!... Don't Push": Motivating Learning in Physics through Student Clubs and Projects." I told you I was a nerd. But don't worry; motivation is way bigger than physics. I got most of my ideas from a book by Deci & Flaste: *Why We Do What We Do: Understanding Self-Motivation*.

There are two types of motivation: *extrinsic* and *intrinsic*. The extrinsic has two forms, the carrot and the stick. We can reward lifters, but you really don't want to pay them to lift. Instead, make clear the result: Power. For a bodybuilder it would be massive size and cuts, being ripped. Keep the right vision in front of your lifters.

How else can you reward lifters for showing up? That's up to you, but most of what works for Monsta are the intrinsic rewards.

Before going there, let's talk about the stick. There are no threats at Monsta. That would be silly. Everything is positive, supporting. Can you picture a room full of meditating monks who get banged on the head with a bamboo stick if their mentor thinks they aren't concentrating? Not at Monsta...but wait, Monsta does have a stick! See the section on *Reps* in the previous chapter. Too many zeros and *follow the leader* continues. Still, you'll see how *follow the leader* also appeals to intrinsic motivation.

Extrinsic motivation comes from outside the lifter. Intrinsic motivation comes from within. Here are components of the gym environment that support a lifter's own desire to lift. They are *choice, challenge,* and *social connection*.

Choice is the easy part. They are there because they want to lift. They choose lifting rather than (or in addition to) running, hiking, climbing, dancing, or cooking. The next three sections will address the need for challenge and social connection.

<u>Two Kinds Of Motivation, Summarized</u>:

- Extrinsic (comes from outside the lifter.), supported by...
    - Carrot = Rewards
    - Stick = Punishment (Don't do this!)
- Intrinsic (comes from inside the lifter.), supported by...
    - Choice
    - Challenge
    - Social Connection

HIERARCHY

In the last section I mentioned that *follow the leader* was extrinsic, but it is more than that because it is a *challenge*. Challenges motivate intrinsically.

Likewise, having a hierarchy among lifters provides a clear and ever present challenge to each lifter. Because of this the hierarchy is motivational. It makes the Monstas try hard with each rep and makes them want to be consistent in attendance.

Each lifter in Monsta gym has a power goal. Mine is to lift 325 lbs. That challenge is attainable, but at my age, I don't see how I will ever get there unless I am tightly focused on that goal. For anyone who has ever attempted a far-off goal, like quitting smoking, saving a certain amount of money, or finding a spouse, he knows how easy it is to get discouraged. Discouragement leads to lapsing. You missed a day not smoking, so you light up the next morning. You needed money, so you might as well skip the *next* month of Roth contributions. That last Match.com date went sour, so you sat the next one out. And so it goes with lifting goals, unless . . .

Unless your big goal is broken into smaller, attainable goals, like knocking the guy in front of you! The Power Guru understands this aspect of human nature, and he works it into the gym. At Monsta, the strongest guy lifts first. Then the next guy goes, etc. As lead spotter, Dan knows where everyone is in the hierarchy, and he knows what they've lifted the last time. He will remind everyone of the order at the start of the workout.

Going up the ladder, guys can warm up with as many reps as they want, but when they get to their working zone, that's where they can knock or be knocked. If a lifter beats the guy in front of him by exceeding his rep count, or if they are tied, but he beats him on the peak weight, he knocks the guy in front of him. Dan allows for one knocking. Everyone can have a bad day. But if the challenger knocks for two workouts in a row, he bumps the guy down a rung in the hierarchy. The next workout, the challenger will be higher than the defeated, who, in turn, will want his place back. (Since this drama might play out over 4 or 5 sets, Dan will consider total rep counts before it becomes clear a knocking has occurred.)

I have both knocked and been knocked up and down the hierarchy, and it does motivate. But we all act like it doesn't! My first knock target was Paul. When I met him I thought to myself, "Why is he above me?" "Is he stronger? He doesn't look like it." (In fact, we have very similar builds, but the ego does get involved.) I remember the day I finally got my first knock. Our working zone weight was 235. I pulled out 7 reps, a rep or two more than Paul. It never resulted in a bumping, because Paul's work commitments changed, and he had to stop coming.

My second knock resulted in a bump. The surprising thing to me was that it was Jonathan I passed. Jonathan looks and is quite a bit bigger than me. He's like a mini-Pete—thick in the shoulders and chest. That position was hard to hold. Jonathan blew past me and is currently repping 325 where I am still doing one, maybe two at 285. Still, the opportunity to get those knocks kept me pushing hard.

My last personal bumping saw me lose a spot. Alex, my son, got me two workouts in a row. I knew the day would come when he would pass me, but I didn't want it to be so soon! This kept me pushing after the knock as hard as it did before the knock. I had to get my spot back.

An interesting note about these three knock experiences: In the months following the knocks, consistency of attendance determined the ultimate positioning in the hierarchy. For example, Paul had to drop out, so his fate was clear. Alex' outside commitments ramped up as well, so his lifting dropped off and I passed him back. Finally, while I have been good about lifting, less of it has occurred at Monsta, whereas Jonathan kept coming and passed me up decisively.

I asked Jason Padgette on his thoughts about the hierarchy.

Burtson:
    Hierarchy, does it motivate?

Padgette:
    Absolutely.

Burtson:
    It's funny, because you've been on top of the hierarchy . . .

Padgette:
    You always want to stay on top and that's the hard part. It's also hard to self motivate when you are on the top. You know you could push more; you know you can do more. You don't have that drive when there's no one right there with you.

Indeed, it's lonely at the top. Jason recognizes the power of the hierarchy. His unique position leaves him without a challenge. Sounds like the next thing to motivate him will have to come from outside the gym, maybe going for a new world record. In fact, he acknowledges there is a record he can pursue one weight class down.

This hierarchy thing has got to be rare in the weight lifting world. Show me a gym where the guys come at the same time on the same two days a week. Show me also a gym where the egos will tolerate getting knocked and bumped. On the contrary—look at *24-Hour Fitness*. Heck, look at the name! It implies coming and going whenever you want. Look at *LA Fitness* for example, where "being fit has never been more flexible." Monsta gym is not about being flexible or being just "fit". It's about being a Monsta, and that takes a little more commitment and *a lot* more challenge.

Hierarchy, Summarized:

- Hierarchy supports intrinsic motivation by providing challenge.
- The strongest guys lift first/ weakest guys last.
- If a challenger exceeds the working zone weight total rep count of the lifter in front of him, he "knocks" him.
- Lead spotter verbally acknowledges the knocks that took place that night, congratulating the knockers.
- Two knocks in a row results in a bump.
- Lifters achieving a bump get placed one spot higher at the next workout.

CAMARADERIE

Without the *camaraderie*, there could be no hierarchy. Who would tolerate it? But we are talking about motivation. How does camaraderie support motivation? Directly. Social connection is one of the three legs of the intrinsic motivation stool. That's camaraderie. Everyone's in it together, all for one, one for all, towards a common goal: power.

And yet *camaraderie* deserves to be more than a subset of something else. The Guru thinks it's the most important thing.

Burtson:
> There is some aspect of what you do that is like the greatest gym on the planet, so if you could bottle it . . .

Fa'asamala:

People try to give me credit for this, but it's the chemistry. It's the camaraderie. I mean, you see these guys. They haven't even met Alex, and they talked about how strong he was, and how well he's adapted to it.

You won't hear too many guys talk about stuff like that, normally when they get together in a group of guys, either they are too macho, or whatever the case might be. But (our guys) watch your progress. You'll notice—no stimulation from me, they'll cheer you on. Because they've watched you come in here and work hard from when you started to where you are right now, and they know because of the work you put in—it motivates them.

What's good about this—though we have a hierarchy—they'll motivate you. But by the same token, they sure wouldn't mind getting in front of you, because if you start doing more weight than the person in front of you, I'll have to move you around, because that's the way it works. It makes it easier for us moving the weights around, and it'll motivate the next guy.

If I'm in front of you and all of a sudden you are doing more weight than I am, I'm going, *Uh oh, he does that again, that's a knock.* We call it a knock. If you get two knocks in a row, and then you've got to switch places. That's just the way it's been.

You are allowed one bad workout, but two? Yeah, no worries, you'll catch up to him if you want, but if not, no biggie. The weights go on.

But the secret or the thing that makes this gym work really well is the camaraderie, the chemistry of the kids that are here. They are here because they want to be here.

This passage captures all the motivational elements: choice ("they want to be here,") challenge, and social connection, but Dan puts the connection part above all the rest. It is his answer to the "greatest gym" question. Furthermore, it takes the focus off him. It's not what he does, he claims, it's the camaraderie. True or not, the Guru sets the tone.

After lifting in the gym for over a year, I continue to be amazed at the environment. Some of the guys are musicians. They are nearly thirty years younger than me, but we talk freely of our common experiences—my history playing live music, my son's goals with his, what style they play, where they are playing, etc. Nothing separates us: tattoos, the clothes we wear, our race, or our age. And when I am benching and I approach a rep count I've never hit before, the shouts start, the encouragements come from every corner of the garage, "C'mon Eric!! You've got it!" So, it's not only Dan who takes notice, but all the Monstas know where you are and what you're after. It is motivational.

Jason is arguably the biggest success story of the garage. Aside from Dan himself, he has been the most consistent. I ask why.

Burtson:
    What make you guys consistent?

Padgette:
    Cameraderie and the love that we have here. Mr. Faas has always been like a father figure to me. He's family basically. He and his sons, we all grew up together. We all treat each other like family. I just enjoy being around him, and coming here and lifting with them.

Last summer, when Joe started coming, it only took him two sessions before declaring it was the highlight of his summer. The story is similar for a lot of these guys. Without camaraderie, Monsta would not be Monsta, and these Monstas would be just men.

But how do you establish camaraderie? What's the recipe? It started from scratch and grew organically. The gym's size expands and shrinks over time. People move; some take on more responsibility. Sometimes people come back, and some never leave. But there is undeniably some draw, some glue that maintains this camaraderie. I speculate.

Personally, I lead two men's groups. In one, we talk about personal issues, usually focused on a book, usually one connected to the men's movement. We meet every other week. Members keep coming because they declare they get a lot out of it—real emotional growth, inspiring us to rise to new challenges.

In the other group, we get together once a month at a sports bar. Over beers we talk about what's going on in our lives, or we just talk. Our stories are usually about our goals, accomplishments, struggles, and hopes. This is what men talk about. It fills a need. It clarifies purpose; it sows seeds for future missions.

Members in both groups do not want to stop meeting. If nothing else, it establishes a truth, that—despite living in a culture that celebrates individualism—men need to be with other men.

Likewise, in a culture where every kid is acknowledged with a trophy, Monsta gym recognizes real achievement. Furthermore, in a culture where decisions are made democratically, and future action dies in a committee, where excitement is snuffed out like wings torn off eagles, Monsta gym has a leader, a leader who encourages you to achieve beyond your dreams, and a leader who helps you get there.

The best word I can use to describe the feel of Monsta Gym is "tribal". It is primordial, yet it is human, very human.

Maybe that's because it has all the motivational elements you could ask for: choice, challenge, and social connection. And let's not forget a leader . . .

Camaraderie, Summarized:

- Camaraderie supports intrinsic motivation as social connection.
- The Guru thinks it is the most important component of a successful gym.
- The Guru sets the example for all other lifters, by participating in every aspect of the gym, from lifting and competing, to congratulating others.
- The Guru establishes a family atmosphere, including acceptance and accountability of all and for all.
- The Guru will ask individuals to leave if they do not support a positive environment.
- The Guru sets goals for himself and gets each lifter to set a personal goal.
- The Guru takes leadership over the proper operation of the gym, from remembering where each lifter is, to enforcing the hierarchy, to congratulating individual achievement.

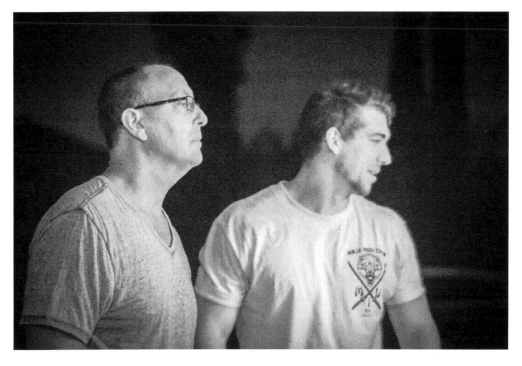

GURU'S PERSONAL REMINDERS

Dan is gracious about people having to miss workouts. He acknowledges that as people get jobs and get married, there are more demands and more time conflicts that have to be resolved one way or the other. He's accepting even when the excuse is weak. A guy who missed a lift texted him, "Yeah sorry, the twelve ounce curl became a lot easier. I got carried away with that". Dan's response was "No worries, the lift went on."

At the same time, he knows the urgency and the importance of not only being consistent, but also being consistent about lifting in Monsta garage. So, he will remind people. His method uses both extrinsic and intrinsic motivation. This is how he does it:

After a work out he might recognize advancement. Or, if a lifter is excited about achieving some new milestone, or regaining something that was lost, Dan will congratulate him. Then, he will say, something like, "Now, imagine if you could be more consistent . . ." Then, in the same breath, he will summon up a particular vision, "Remember when you were repping 325, how good that felt? You can get there much quicker." Or, "Look at Pete, what a Monster! He used to be so skinny . . ."

This is extrinsic, because he's asking. And, because his Monstas love him, it compels them to comply. But he also makes it intrinsic by pulling up a vision. They are in it because they want to be, and he reminds them of that reason.

Furthermore, though he might project an image of being relaxed about this, he isn't. It's too important. He might say, "If you guys don't show up, that tempts me to go back in my room and play my games." (In other words, no big deal, I've got other things to do, but you also help me out by showing up.) The reality is that Dan is on the lookout for how to most effectively deliver that message, so much that it happens at almost every workout. And, while he might be directing it to one person in particular, everyone hears it.

Here's an example of Dan extending himself to motivate others. My son Alex was with me during my first interview for this book. When I asked my first question, Dan turned it around and asked Alex how he was feeling after the workout. He proceeded to give Alex feedback about how quickly he was coming along, and how pleased he was to see it. Then, a few pages into the interview, he told Alex the story of Peter, how Peter was so super skinny when he started and how strong he is now, and how his consistency got him there.

Here is a final point on the importance of the Guru's reminders. Dan doesn't like it when I call this the best gym on the planet. Who would? It puts a lot of pressure on you to maintain that image — it's a big burden. I do that because I believe it, but I believe it in a very specific way: that it is the most effective at building bench power naturally. And yet it is obvious that Dan values a workout here in Monsta gym far above anything a person might do outside the garage. This implies he knows he has something special going here, that there is some magic about this place. He might not call it the best gym, but he knows it's far superior to other venues. Furthermore, if he is going to make world champions, there needs to be some level of intensity and commitment, otherwise, it's just a club. And Dan won't settle for that, because he's not just a club president, he's a Guru.

<u>Guru's Personal Reminders, Summarized:</u>

- Give a low-pressure appeal for more frequent attendance. Combine this with a reminder of the lifter's goal. This will motivate consistent lifting.
- Direct these reminders to individual lifters, as they experience success.
- Don't be shy about others hearing.
- Always look for opportunities to encourage in this way.

6. Guru Coaching

On my very first visit last year, long before any formal interviews, I sat with Dan. In a casual conversation he told me what he thought most distinguished his garage from other gyms: his spotting style. That's what this whole chapter is about.

When you see the phrase *"lead spotter,"* I mean Dan and the way he does things. His lead spotter work carries the bulk of what makes him a guru. Being a guru is leading, applying a vast reserve of technical knowledge and wisdom, and coaching. You'll see that throughout this chapter.

Dan's leadership and his coaching are such a part of Monsta that I couldn't help writing about them in earlier chapters, but here we will focus on this. I am convinced that without Dan, these men might have become animals at best, but never Monstas.

SAFE IS SEXY

Also on that first day Dan said the only thing he prays for before a workout is safety. "No one gets hurt on my watch," he says. Of course no one wants to get hurt at a workout. It doesn't help your lifting progress either.

I used to lift without a spotter. Once, doing the CGSG, the bar slid out of my left hand. It was well over two hundred pounds, and fortunately, I was able to catch it on my forearm. It stripped off a little skin, maybe left a little strawberry wound, but I could live with it. However, if I had suffered a pull during my lift, without a proper spot it might have become a full tear, setting me back months. I would rather deal with a strawberry burn than four months of missed progress.

It is especially heartbreaking when a big guy gets injured. As I mentioned above, the body is efficient, it will only keep muscle tissue if it needs it. Once you get past a certain size and strength, the gains don't come easily. You are fighting with your body to keep those gains. You turn off the stimulation and your body starts to devour itself. Therefore it is well worth the boredom of plodding through a number of "meaningless" low-weight warms-ups if they prevent you from big self-cannibalization losses.

Therefore, if you want to be pushing really big weights, you've got to stop taking a step back for every two forward. Sooner or later you'll be taking one step back for every step forward, and you'll be going nowhere. This is why safe *is* sexy.

Joe is an example of how an injury can set you back. He had only been coming for three months when he had a weekend jackhammer accident. It was a nerve pinch, but it made his muscles weak, and affected his form. He still kept lifting with light weights, but by the time he healed, nine months had passed. At the end of those months he finally returned to his former strength, but all that opportunity for progress had passed. Happily, he has made strong gains in the past two months, pushing him to new personal records at almost every session. Without commitment like Joe's and the motivating environment of the gym, I do not believe many people would have kept coming back through a similar ordeal.

It is interesting to note that over the last year and a quarter most of the standard pinches and stiffness I've seen in these lifters came from outside the gym. The ladder, the emphasis on stretching and warming with low weights—all these procedures are responsible for keeping injuries to a minimum.

Usually, the physical complaints are trivial enough to allow the lifter to participate in the workout. Dan makes the call. He asks the lifter to be honest about any injury up front. Then he asks for updates on pain throughout the workout. At times, he'll say, "You're done today, go rest." At other times, he'll keep the weight small. Sometimes he just monitors, but the workout is unaffected. The lifter retains the joy of going heavy.

Dan's personal story about the importance of safety is painfully compelling. Just a couple or few years ago Dan was competing in a local bench press competition. After warm-ups it was clear to him he was going to win. Still continuing with his warm-ups, he put on 450 lbs. This was quite a bit less than his target lift for the day, but he noticed the crowd was already engaged. This motivated him to trivialize the weight, so he attempted to pop it up quickly off his chest. Then something went terribly wrong.

He felt three hard tugs in his left pec. He was done for the day. When he took it to the doctor, the doctor explained that Dan had completely torn three major cords in his chest. The muscle was now bunched up near the joint. Reconnecting it was out of the question, as it would require cutting through a lot of other muscle to get to the fix.

The injury was painful, and it ended any hope of competing again. He prayed. It took months before he could lift the bar. He continued to pray. It took equally long before he could lift a bar and a plate. But somehow he was able to bring it back to repping over 400 lbs. Safety matters.

<u>Safe is Sexy, Summarized:</u>

- Stretch before lifting.
- Observe the slow ladder warm up in every lifting situation, inside or outside the gym.
- Don't risk being injured outside the gym unless you like taking risks or your job requires it.
- If you have a muscular injury, however minor, share it with the coach.
- Coach, monitor the injured person's pain through the workout and use common sense in guiding him through a modified workout.
- If you are injured, persevere. Lift conservatively if you can, but resume fully as soon as you are healed.

LIGAMENTS AND TENDONS

Remember running away as a kid? You got mad at your folks. You were feeling your oats. You showed them. You got up and left.

There comes a time when kids get good at moving around and finding places to hide. These are big steps on the way to adulthood. But what they don't realize is they have no bank account and no income. It won't take too long before their forward progress screeches to a halt. They lack the supporting structures.

So it is with muscles. Dan preaches on the importance of building *the house*, which is the combination of your ligaments and tendons and muscles. He believes your initial growth in muscle size can pass the accommodations in the supporting tissues, resulting in possible tears, strains, and pulls.

Moreover, he believes that further muscle growth *must be preceded* by growth in the ligaments and tendons.

Therefore, to protect his lifters and to get them ready for the next big gains, he works the fringes, the ligaments and tendons.

You see this most dramatically when a new lifter comes to the gym. He will make him do light weights, sometimes for several workouts. This not only allows Dan to concentrate on developing the lifter's form, but it prepares the ligaments and tendons.

So, you might see a guy come in with the ability to bench 250 lbs, but he ends up going no higher than single plates. This could be frustrating for a newbie who wants to show he's one of the guys, but that's the way it has to be.

For the rest of the lifters, sticking with the low-weight start of the Monsta ladder helps maintain strength in the ligaments and tendons.

To prepare a lifter for a max never before achieved, Dan will make sure the lifter has acquired the ability to maintain excellent form at a high weight near the pending max. He will also look for an increased number of reps at that weight before he will trust the lifter with the new peak weight. He's looking for a thumbs-up from the ligaments and tendons.

Ligaments and Tendons, Summarized:

- Keep doing the Monsta ladder, starting at low weights
- Have new lifters in the gym spend a couple or few workouts handling weight much under their ability to lift.
- Work on the new lifter's form during this low weight phase.
- Assure him you are doing this to build his form and the foundation of the surrounding tissues.
- Prepare an established lifter for his new peak weight by dwelling at a slightly lower weight for several workouts, maintaining good form and increasing the rep count.

TRIPLE SPOT

Dan's commitment to safety doesn't mean he takes no chances. As Machiavelli says, "Never was anything great achieved without danger." Consider the name of Monsta's staple lift, *close grip with suicide grip*. I asked Jason about it. You already know he thinks it is effective, but safety was an issue.

Burtson:
    What do you think of the *close grip with suicide grip*?

Padgette:
    I love it now. It used to be my weak lift, and I have to admit, the first time I ever did it, I felt unsafe.

    After doing it a number of years, I've never had any accidents with it. And I've been doing it for 16 years now. The bar has never slipped out of my hands. It's never rolled out, or bounced off my chest.

With Dan spotting, the bar is not likely to bounce off anyone's chest, that is, until the weight gets real heavy. When lifters combine the CGSG with anything over 300 pounds, that hikes up the risk.

Dan knows that if he's going to let his boys play with fire, he's going to have a fire hose in the gym. That fire hose is the *triple spot*.

The rule is that whenever anyone lifts over 300 pounds, the other strongest three lifters arrange themselves around the bar. Dan goes directly over the lifter, in the lead spotting position he always holds. The others go to the two ends of the bar. And they pay attention.

If a lifter needs a little help getting that last rep up, Dan will give a finger assist. The two side spotters know not to touch the bar unless there is an accident. All it takes is one overly enthusiastic side spotter, and his lone intervention creates a dangerous situation of its own.

Once in a while I'm high enough in the lift order that I am supposed to do spot duty. But I usually forget. By the time I notice, the next guy down the hierarchy has already stepped around me and taken a side position. These guys are trained and aware.

Triple Spot, Summarized:

- When anyone lifts over three hundred pounds, the top three lifters in the hierarchy snap to the triple spot position.
- The triple spot keeps the lead spotter in the lead spotter position, unless the lead spotter is lifting.
- Only the lead spotter (in the center position, over the lifter) assists on any reps.
- Side spotters do not touch the bar, except when an accident has occurred or if the lead spotter gives the order.
- All spotters pay careful attention and stay ready to act.

TRUST AND THE LEAD SPOTTER'S WORK FOR EACH LIFTER

Dan never gives up his lead spotting role. I used to think it was because he was the strongest lifter. He can dead lift 800 pounds, which is a comforting thought. But depending on who's there, he's not always the strongest. Dan keeps the lead spot because that's where he does most of his coaching.

The most important part of his coaching is earning the lifter's trust. It's a physical and psychological investment in getting the lifter to believe he can safely lift anything the lead spotter puts on the bar. He explains it best.

Burtson:
    Explain the psychology of the spot.

Fa'asamala:

It's like anything else; it's relationship. Guys come in here and they lift, some guys come from wherever. I have to get their trust, and how do I do that? I spot. I'll put weight on there that they normally wouldn't put on their own. I take them through regimes, like twelve or fourteen sets. So they're pretty beat up. They wouldn't do [that] on their own. A lot of these guys, even Jason, he wouldn't work out as hard as he does work out if I didn't push him. But they all know; if I put it on there, I'll make sure they get it off.

Pete. . .he pretty much trusts me with his life. If I put four or five hundred pounds on that bar, he might look at me, but he'll say, "Ok, if you say so!" He'll get under that bar, and he'll go ahead and push. Whether he gets it off the arms or not he'll push, because he trusts me that much.

Like you, when you first came, you trusted my heart from the beginning, but over time, you'll notice you'll push more, you'll probably do more weight, and go for more reps then you normally would on your own, right?

And building a relationship with a spotter, when you go to a gym, you might have somebody spot you, but that's a once in a lifetime thing. You don't know when that guy's going to show up again, You don't know what kind of spotter he is. So while you're thinking about all that stuff, you're still trying to get your weight.

Where with me, and the consistency of the relationship; you know exactly what my expectations are; you know exactly how I am going to spot. And you know I'm going to let you do most of the work anyways. You'll get to a point where I'll see in your body, where, *Ok, I'm just going to take it off you*, but I won't jerk it off you. I'll push it off, tap it off you.

You've seen it. Some guys you ask for a spot, and they pull it right off. Well, that sort of messes the happy, happy end to my expectations I had . . .
You want to finish off the rep, and somebody just takes it off.

Or you'll have somebody put the hands on the weight the whole time. I don't need you to be all that. We talked about the . . . philosophy, based on what my father taught me – *You can't pick it up, you don't touch it.*

Early in my participation of Monsta garage, I was impressed by Dan's interactions with his guys, and by how hard those guys pushed. Being the science guy I am, I tried to reduce the whole thing to an equation. Dan doesn't like the equation, and neither do I anymore: There is too much to capture in one phrase. That's why there's this book. However, I still think there's merit to stating this relationship:

    Commitment to the person
\+ promise of safety
\+ promise of success (positive vision with no downside)
= Lifter's exertion   = Muscle growth

It's not just exertion either. As Dan said, "You will lift more weight for more reps than you would on your own."

The guys often talk about why it is they can lift more in this gym than anywhere else. Is it the motivating music? Is it all the guys being there? Is it Faas' coaching? Truth is, that's probably the biggest reason. If nothing else, the guru's demonstrated commitment flips a switch in the lifter's attitude making him go absolutely balls out.

Trust And The Lead Spotter's Work For Each Lifter, Summarized:

- The Lead Spotter has a reputation for being strong.
- The Lead Spotter is engaged in every rep of every set for each lifter.
- The Lead Spotter speaks encouragement to the lifter.
- The Lead Spotter does not yank the weight off a spent lifter. He applies just enough force to let the lifter complete the rep on his own.
- At each lifter's peak lift, the lead spotter puts a weight the lifter would likely not attempt on his own.
- At times, the lead spotter will prescribe exactly how many reps he wants to see the lifter achieve.

LEAD SPOTTER KNOWLEDGE OF LIFTERS' STRENGTHS

I was going to call this section "Lead Spotter Sets Targets," but that doesn't quite catch what Dan does. This incident explains:

A couple of weeks ago, eighteen guys showed up to lift. A couple of them were new. As the four-minute stretch time was coming to an end, Dan was at his normal position behind the bar. He was leaning over the bar with a furrowed brow, trying to see who was there, inside and outside the garage. I saw him mouth the names of the lifters, "Jason," "Big Jon," etc. He was establishing the hierarchy for the day.

He was basing his ranking on his knowledge of the lifters' working ranges. One of the lifters had just returned from a not-too-short absence. He positioned him about six guys below where he was last, based on his understanding of how much he probably lost being gone so long. Dan was really close with his estimation. He also had to work in the new guys. Usually, he asks them how much weight they train with. That helps.

Dan's knowledge of the lifter is much more detailed than where each one is relative to the other lifters. He knows what you are working on, and he knows what you're ready for. We had a discussion about my progress:

Burtson:
>The last time I lifted, you limited me to two reps with two plates, saying, *I want you to feel your power*. Then you loaded it to 285. You were managing me personally. Do you do this with all the guys?

Fa'asamala:
>I do. If you'll notice, everybody has a time. I'll condition you, and get you ready mentally, physically. Then . . . when I have you pushing two plates, you could probably do four reps . . . but I was noticing your strokes are lot more even; there's more foundation in the way you push. So I just want you to get used to that.
>
>Especially in your head I want you to look at that bar and know, "*This thing is moving.*" And you have a better foundation. So I'm conditioning you mentally and physically. It's not a physical issue for you anymore.
>Now I've got to get you mentally ready to jump next time.
>
>And then you'll hear me say, when you're hitting heavier weight, 285 or so, *Get used to it*, because you'll be pushing on that a lot more.

Burtson:
>That's close to 300.

Fa'asamala:
>Yeah, but that's not gonna be the end.

Dan being able to hold that much info in his head — to me it seems that's a special gift. Knowing what the lifter is ready for even before the lifter knows it — that's uncanny. Being able to condition the lifter's psychological state — that's guru status.

At this point in the book you are probably thinking how you might adapt some of what Dan does so that you don't have to actually be a guru to get world-class results. I encourage your adaptations. Here is one idea. Rather than trying to remember where each person is, have a large white board in the gym. Have all the guys listed. Have four columns: Current repping weight, current max, short-term max goal, long term max goal. From there, it's a snap to set the hierarchy regardless of who shows up. Also, if they are not ready to have their numbers posted, that's a sign they don't yet have enough trust. If no one wants it posted, the camaraderie is not there yet.

Lead Spotter's Knowledge of Lifters' Strengths, Summarized:
- The Lead Spotter knows each lifter's current repping weight and personal goals.
- The Lead Spotter anticipates when the lifter is ready for a move up.
- The Lead Spotter discerns when a plateau is purely mental.
- The Lead Spotter challenges the lifter with weights he knows the lifter can handle.
- The Lead Spotter might want to write this information on a white board.

LEAD SPOTTER'S UNQUESTIONED REGIMEN

One of my least favorite things to do is work for a boss who micromanages. I need freedom to try ideas and to pursue those that work. That's why I'm currently happier working for my own investment adviser business than for the "established" company I used to work for. I want the possibility of bigger gains.

And that's exactly what Dan has done in over thirty years of experimenting in his garage. When something is shown to work so well for so long someone needs to write down the process. Voilà.

Now that the process is shown to produce world-class results, it deserves respect. Doubtless, it will be experimented with, and it should, but the maker and his disciples should revel in the structure they have. Dan is justified in his assertions.

It also helps to take direction from someone who cares about you. I do believe, at his command, his guys would march into the ocean wearing full sets of armor.

I questioned Dan about other methods. He told me a story about a guy who trained multiple muscle groups using four or five different lifts per group, and who ran four or five miles a day. He asked Dan for his advice, but didn't take it:

Fa'asamala:
>(The guy said,) *Uncle Danny, I've been working out like 5 times a week, but I just can't get the size!* He's one of those kids who, if he stuck around . . . sheesh, he would have been doing really, really well.
>
>He's got all kinds of stuff going on in his life, so . . .You're not resting your muscles . . . The secret of the workout is the rest. If you don't let your body rest, you're not giving it enough time to grow like you want it to grow.

Burtson:
>Would you say running interferes with it?

Fa'asamala:
> Well, you're breaking down muscle. That's the overall body breaker. If you're running 4 or 5 miles, you're not giving your body the rest it needs . . . If you're working out for endurance, yes. What he wants, he wants to look buff, go to the beach, look a little GQ. That's really not what I'm giving you. I'm here to make you strong. That other stuff is a side effect of what we do. That's what I call the Captain America workout, you'll get stronger, but you won't get the results you are looking for.

In interviews and in real life situations I've witnessed him repeat the same message: You can do it differently, but you won't make the same gains. What you want determines what you do. At Monsta, we want power.

That's the same message my son got when Dan found out he was training at cross-fit. It's the same message I got when I said I was going vegan. It's the same message anyone would get if they said they wanted to add squats to the workout.

Once, my workout was a little off. As I was coming off the bench Dan asked, "So how's that Vegan diet working out?" Then he turned to Jonathan (one up in the rankings) and asked, "Where did you eat today Jonathan?" Jonathan answered, "In-n- Out".

However, none of this is really micromanagement. Dan lets you do whatever you want. Recently, one of the lifters brought a preacher curl bench into the garage. It was there for months. Some of the guys used it between sets. Dan even showed them how to use it properly, but if you asked him, he'd say it takes away.

Michi Takeda (see *Vision*, below) compares Dan to other leaders she has trained under. She remembers one man in particular who had a reputation for being totally inflexible. Though Dan believes in his technique, Dan always "gave people the opportunity to find out" for themselves. Ninety percent of the time they would realize Danny was right anyway. This was one of the reasons Michi liked training under Dan. She drove 100 miles round trip from Irvine twice a week, just to be at Monsta Garage.

Going back to the discussion on unquestioned regimen, it might seem silly that we are extracting so much from one lift. In reality, there is a lot to Guru Fa'samala's methods: the two grips, safety, constant tension, consistency, the hierarchy, trust—everything mentioned above. I personally hope people use these methods in their purest form. I want to see these people push the envelope and break more records. I even hope they experiment and improve the process, but I fully believe it has to start here, Monsta-style.

<u>Lead Spotter's Unquestioned Regimen, Summarized:</u>

- Do the method and the method only. Any additional exercise competes for the rest needed by the targeted muscles.
- If you want other things like leg development or cardio conditioning, add them to your training, but know that they will take away from upper body power.
- After making good progress with these methods, feel free to experiment, but please report back any perceived improvements.

LEAD SPOTTER'S ACTIVE VERBAL COMMANDS AND ENCOURAGEMENTS

Two sections ago, I explained that Dan maintains a mental record of not only the weight each lifter is working with, but the weight each lifter is ready for. He also knows the psychology of each lifter. This comes out in what he says to the lifter during the set. He says two kinds of things. One set of sayings simply directs what the lifter does. The other set encourages the lifter.

The first kind is pretty standard, "I want you to do three more reps," "Come up higher," "Start a little lower on the chest," "Don't jerk; bring it down smooth," or "Put it away."

These are important for a couple of reasons: First, so the lifter can employ proper mechanics and to gain optimal stimulation; second, to let the lifter know he is important, and gets the guru's full attention.

The second kind of statement Dan gives is meant to encourage. Some lifters—some of the biggest, strongest, longest lifting lifters—actually don't like pushing the weights. While I personally enjoy benching, I don't like squatting. If you put over two hundred pounds on a squat bar, add your body to that, and go deep, that's lifting over four hundred pounds through a large stroke. It is painful and exhausting. I've known people to almost black out after a set of squats. Ask a woman why giving childbirth is so infamously painful, and she might tell you it's because of those uncontrollable, deep, vice-like contractions of that giant internal uterus muscle. Once you are repping 400 pounds on the bench, it's probably the closest a man gets to that kind of struggle. That's probably why by the end of the workout the top three lifters are dripping with sweat while the other guys are still dancing around. For these exhausted strongmen Dan will often say to the whole gym, "This is a light day," or "We're almost there, just one more set!" Then there's everyone's favorite: "I promise you, your competition . . . is at home eating a Twinkie!"

To newer lifters, or those who seem nervous or hurried, he'll frequently say, "This is your time," or "You're the only one on that bench. This is for you, not anyone else."

Dan has a lot of things to say to the discouraged, or to those who doubt they can reach their goals. Some of these people need to know that they are capable of moving weight. He'll often say, "Get a good feel." Sometimes Dan will put a big weight on the bar and say, "I just want you to get one strong rep with good form and put it away."

Other times he will appeal to that fire deep inside, "Big heart". He often teases, "Do you really wanna be that strong?" But my favorite of Dan's expressions is what he says to someone who just made a breakthrough. Maybe they've just lifted a weight they've been trying to get for a long time, or maybe they didn't really think they could do it. As the lifter ratchets the bar past the toughest part of the push, he'll say, "Well how about that."

In response the lifter might bounce off the bench beaming, "I can't believe I did that!" to which Dan will reply, "Get used to it, because you're going to be pushing that a lot more . . . and that's not gonna be the end." So, just as the lifter achieves a goal he was unsure he could ever hit, Dan confidently asserts he will see more gains. As a result, with each breakthrough the lifter starts to believe more in what Dan says, and less in his own doubts.

When seven, eight or eighteen people show for a lift, that leaves a lot of downtime. But that's not a problem. It's more like a party. People interact, laugh and talk. Sometimes we analyze how our lifting is going. We all agree that when Dan says one of these things to us—though we might have heard him say it before—it always seems fresh and sincere.

Lead Spotter's Active Verbal Commands And Encouragements, Summarized:

- The Lead Spotter gives lifters technical/mechanical feedback; coach during the lift.
- The Lead Spotter encourages lifters in order to address their
    - Exhaustion
    - Feelings of insignificance
    - Discouragement
    - Disbelief

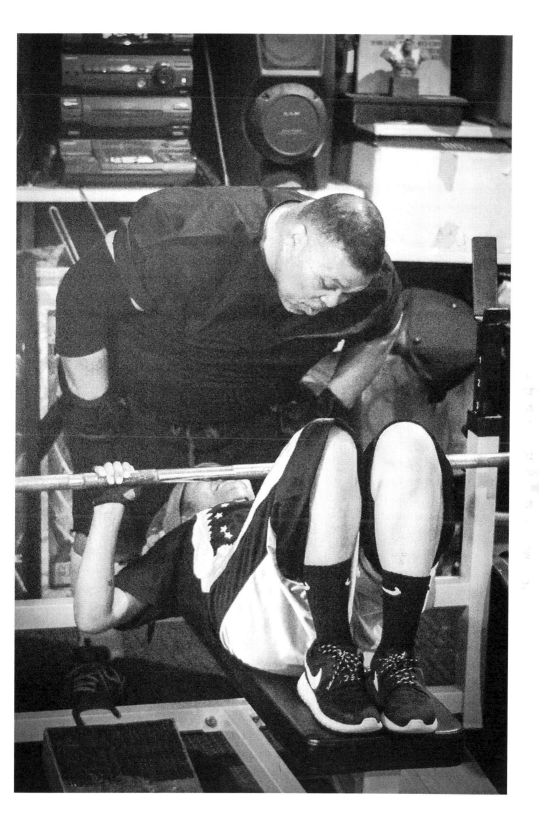

LEAD SPOTTER'S MUTUAL PARTICIPATION

Dan recently had surgery. It wasn't minor. The doctor told him not to lift for about three months. If my memory serves me, it ended up being two workouts. Even on those two days, Dan was still in the gym.

After that, he was back in position as lead spotter. The lead spotter is the most active person in the gym. The second most active is the guy at the top of the hierarchy. These two are so busy because they have to swap weights out to accommodate each lifter.

Usually two or three lifters in a row use the same weight, but at several points through the round of lifters the spotters need to take off 25s or 45s. Then they reload everything when the top of the order comes back around. Dan was doing all that about one week after his surgery.

He could easily have another main guy take the other end of the bar and swap out weights. He could just concentrate on coaching from the middle. But he feels it is essential that he work harder than anyone in the gym. That way, he says, no one can claim to be overtired or overworked. Incidentally Dan's also the eldest guy in the gym (uh, by a few days).

Moreover, Dan's not just being a good example; he genuinely loves lifting. Earlier this month, a certain song came on the playlist. Dan was pumped, saying, "I can't wait for it to be my turn. It's gotta be my turn."

Lead Spotter's Mutual Participation, Summarized:

- The Lead Spotter sets the example by working as hard or harder than any other lifter.
- The Lead Spotter lifts when everyone else lifts. He doesn't have to lift more than everyone; he just lifts hard with them.
- The Lead Spotter shows his enthusiasm for lifting.

THE LEAD SPOTTER'S VISION

When I started lifting at Monsta I thought I would give a survey to all the guys, then compare their results to what other lifters say:

> Why do you lift? Is it A) for health, B) to look good, C) to feel good, D) for fun, or E) to get powerful?

I quickly learned the survey wasn't necessary. At Monsta, it's all about the power. "I want you to feel your power" is another expression Dan will often say. Dan uses the word *power* frequently, and I think intentionally. Each lifter's peak lifting weight is a measure of that power, and it's always on everyone's mind.

Dan uses power as a gauge for progress. And it's not always just about how much you lift or how many reps you do. For him it's more about how much you do under conditions of control. Here's what he says:

Burtson:
>How Important is form?

Fa'asamala:
>Technique, that's everything. I don't care how much weight you can push. You've seen how many times you'll see these guys get in the gym. They'll throw like three plates on; they'll arch their back, they'll have crooked elbows; one side comes up before the other; put it away and they make claim to that. Ok, you say you did get it up—ugly as it may be. But ever since we started real competition, technique and power (became important).
>
>We were introduced to the pause rep, where they bring the bar down; you hold it there until the bar is steady; then the judge says "press". You won't understand the control of power until you've done that one time.
>
>When we were introduced to that, that made me understand, that's power. You could sit there and rep it all day, but you are taking advantage of rhythm, —from dead stop, yeah, that's impressive; that's nothing but you.

But what is power, and why would anyone want it? You've heard the expression *money is power*. Turn it around to make it *power is money*. In a sense, they are equivalent. Each is a currency, a commodity, a quantity of value. But so are *health, wisdom, intelligence, time, relationships* and *creativity*. Why would anyone want any of these? Who wouldn't want all of these? And who can have all of these? The best example is Solomon. He asked for wisdom, so the LORD gave him everything. Now, I'm not sure that Solomon could bench press very much, but he had an army and angels to back him up.

These are foolish questions, because as humans, we are all in pursuit of value. Even Buddhist monks are looking for peace, they just look for a direct way to peace that doesn't depend on first having any of the other commodities.

But if life is a smorgasbord of choices, the Monstas make room for a sizeable portion of physical power on their plates. What value do they get from it?   Before I show you Dan's answer, I brainstormed a list. As an exercise you might want to brainstorm a list yourself, though I imagine if you are reading this book you already know why power is useful.

My uses of power:

- Fighting to defend others or myself
- Keeping the peace
- Having peace of mind
- Lifting cars off people
- Getting out from under rubble
- Tossing kids in the air
- Getting lids off jars
- Combat
- Defense against road rage
- Stopping dog attacks
- Slugging muggers
- Helping people move

For example, last weekend my wife invited her friend over. She brought her two daughters and one of their friends. I tried to interest the three of them in being tossed in the water. My wife was floating next to me, so, as an example of the fun they were in for, I grabbed her and tossed her up in the air a couple of times. The girls were too little to trust me with that.

Instead, when I was out of the pool, I got the net and extended the handle end of the pole into the pool just above the water. I told one of them to grab on for a tour of the pool. One of the girls latched on, and I walked her from end to end. It was like she was flying through the water. Eventually, they all got a tour. They loved it.

It couldn't have happened without power. That was a long pole. The torque it created on my upper body could not have been matched unless I had power. Most guys wouldn't have thought of the pole tour. Without having the capacity, why would they even think it?

Yes, it's a silly example, but that last sentence can be generalized. *Without having the capacity, why would they even think it?* Having power makes you more capable; it broadens possibilities.

Physical power also has a positive feedback loop. When you train, your body generates more testosterone. The testosterone makes you more powerful. It also gives you confidence. Confidence makes you try more weight. More weight builds more power, and so on.

But confidence also has general purposes. It boosts your likelihood of taking chances in life. It eases interactions on and off work. It makes you more powerful in general. *Health, wisdom, intelligence,* and *creativity* can also boost your confidence, but, as I have shown, so does having physical power.

Here's a practical example: A young woman named Michi Takeda came to Monsta Gym for Dan's help back in 2002 . She was a devoted student of the *Kendo* fighting style, but her lack of power limited her progress. Kendo makes no gender distinctions. Men and women compete in the same tournament.

She remembers one match in particular. A woman used a stall move by trying to stay in close. Michi could not easily push her out where she could score points. Since Michi was trying to qualify for the International Kendo championships, so she knew she had to do something about getting stronger.

When she came to Monsta, she could only lift the bar, 55 pounds. Within nine months she was repping 145 lbs. That strength gave her what she needed. She is now a third degree black belt.

As I promised, here are Dan's thoughts on the advantages of physical power. I was interviewing him when the discussion turned to the effort needed to do this training. Dan said,

You guys drive here from San Diego and you put in the time, 45 minutes to an hour, but that's 45 min to an hour of investment to your body. That's maybe two hours a week you are putting into your selves, that only has to work *one time* — for whatever significant reason. It might even be to lift a car off a loved one or other. That *one time* will make all that investment in time you guys put-in in a week, worth it. That *one time* when you run into somebody who shouldn't have said what he said, and you do what you're supposed to do. And that *one time* when you run into a wall and you go, *Sheesh, I wasn't ready for this!* Uh, you could have been.

Of course, Dan's point of view is somewhat influenced by his career, especially the bodyguard work. He needs access to physical power more than that *one time*, but he understands the value to all of us. We happily buy life insurance and health insurance, maybe for that *one time*. Why not invest in personal power?

Dan acknowledges that power can be a problem. It has been said that power corrupts, and absolute power corrupts absolutely. Dan is on the lookout. I refer to a quote made earlier in the book:

> When you start working with 300 lbs, or 200 lbs actually, you become dangerous. There are expectations I have. I definitely don't want to hear that you are a bully. We don't train bullies. We eat bullies.

If you're going to eat bullies, you'd better be powerful.

The Lead Spotter's Vision, Summarized:

- The Lead Spotter makes it clear that physical power is the training goal.

- The Lead Spotter frequently and intentionally uses the word *power*.
- The Lead Spotter reminds lifters of their lifting goals.
- The Lead Spotter has reasons why power is valuable, and he reminds lifters of these reasons.

LEAD SPOTTER'S LOVE

The first time I interviewed Dan I asked him the best gym question right off the bat.

Burtson:
    Is this the best gym on the planet?

Fa'asamala:
    I don't know about that. When you say best gym in the planet—it's like raising your kids, if love is at the basis of your decision, everything you make, then yeah, but best gym. . .it's great for me, and the boys think so too, that's why they come back.

A quarter hour later we were talking about those seven American and five world champion records. Still interviewing, I asked:

Burtson:
    That's what I'm trying to tease out; what do you do differently?

Fa'asamala:
    I think it's like raising kids. If your basis for raising kids is love, then no matter what decisions you've made, I don't think you can be wrong.

    In this garage anything we do is a benefit to the garage.

> I don't think there is an advantage to me teaching any other style. I'm not trying to gain anything from it. As you know, I don't charge.

Burtson:
> What's the push for this?

Fa'asamala:
> Guys like Roger Metz and you gave to us — gave to me, and it's my way to pay back.
>
> If we had more guys like that nowadays that we had back there for us Eric — Roger Metz is a fine example — imagine how much better this place could be.
>
> If you know anything about Roger Metz, he pretty much raised me and (you) Eric — in the bodybuilding aspect and lifting.
>
> This guy took us out to dinner. This guy took us in and gave us jobs. This guy trained us. He hooked us up with seminars that people would pay megabucks to see. But we saw them, and we became part of the family.
>
> We went to eat at Filipe's right after the competition. We'd help with the gym, the setup, the music, whatever it was. He got us involved. He kept us busy, kept us out of trouble.
>
> If we had maybe one out of twenty — one out of every fifty even — people like that, I think we would be in a better place, a different frame of mind.

I find it interesting that when I put that big question out there about the value and effectiveness of the gym, I got love as the answer. I pressed again and got the same answer. I pressed *again*, and I got detail.

Dan talked about payback. But I don't recall Roger's caring actions as pay of any kind, just pure goodness. I do look back fondly on those days, those experiences, those opportunities that Roger and his wife Jaye gave us. And over this past year, as I've been in the midst of this gym, Dan's care flows just as naturally. It's not pay-back, pay-forward, or pay-anything; it is love.

This past year I got one of my biggest compliments ever. I was teaching physics, walking around the classroom, when a student in the back of the room said, "Mr. Burtson, you're a good teacher, because this other teacher I had didn't care about you if you weren't good in the subject. But you take just as much time with all the kids, no matter how good they are."

I was glad to hear this, because it wasn't always true for me. For too long I was more concerned about test scores. I felt this tremendous pressure to get them up. This had two effects on my action. First, I'm sure I tried harder with the best students because I knew their results would have the most influence on the scores. Second, I was too tense in class. I pushed too hard, and rarely relaxed enough to be a helpful presence away from the white board. The high achievers didn't need me to be among the seats so much, but the strugglers did, and I wasn't there.

Now I understand that each student cares. If they aren't super-engaged with the subject, they still want to be there. They want to pass. They want to graduate. Some of the low performers are just as enthusiastic as anyone, but dyslexia or some other learning limitation makes it hard on them. I don't think of myself as a touchy-feely guy, but I care about them because they care. They matter. Well, ok, it also helps that California isn't testing this year.

That same idea carries over into the gym: care because they care. Everyone matters, school-smart or not, strong or just starting out. During the second interview, I asked a question that got the longest uninterrupted response from Dan. It ended with this story:

Burtson:
>Does the method work automatically, or do you optimize it by this personalization?

Fa'asamala:
>. . . I just could not say no. There was this one kid. He said something to me that blessed my heart forever-and-a-day, and I'll never forget it. He was one of the kids who was always in trouble in school, probably was the guy that talked you into doing something you weren't supposed to do.
>
>But he wanted to hang out with us because he said it was cool. And then he came and started lifting, and he saw the way we were gelling.
>
>My boys came to me and said, *Hey Dad, I don't know about this one.*

I said, *Here's the thing: If he does something I don't like, then I'll let him go, I'll talk to him. But other than that right now he shows up; he lifts. He doesn't give me a hard time; he shows me respect — we're good to go.*

Two months later, after being around this, his mom came by and wanted to watch us lift. I said, *How are you doing? Nice to meet you.*

She said, *Yeah, I just wanted to meet you. My son has been doing well at school, and has been respectful in the house. And he said it has something to do with his lifting.*

I said, *Oh, wow.*

I said, *How about that?*

I was looking at my boys, *How about that? Go figure, he's doing well, huh?* He even brought his brother down.

They ended up moving to the East Coast. He used to call and text me. He showed me pictures of his garage. He said because of our garage, he started a garage over there.

So this kid turned out to be heaven-sent, and he said this to me:
Coming to your garage and lifting with you on Mondays, Wednesdays and Fridays was like having Christmas every Monday, Wednesday and Friday.

I said, *a better compliment a guy could never ask for — Christmas three times a week.* So I said, *Good; go stretch.*

It is interesting to note that there is rarely a conversation that goes like this, "Let's gear up to take some more world records! Let's do this! Let's do thiiiiiis!" Whenever it's mentioned, it's more casual, incidental, almost an afterthought: "We don't have a competition coming up, so we're going to focus more on the close grip." Jason mentioned that he could drop a little bit of weight and take a record, as long as he didn't lose any strength. Maybe he'll do that. Jordan is another guy who is within striking distance of a 135-pound weight class record. I've heard it mentioned, but usually I'm the guy trying to psyche him up for it, and even then it comes off more playful than urgently opportunistic.

So, if the focus is not on the records, and yet records do come, what is the focus? We know that power is the vision. Maybe love is the mission.

It is also interesting to note the special fondness Dan has for the guys who have been coming for fifteen or more years, the Petes, Big Johns, and Jasons of the gym. At the same time, there is no favoritism. No one is forgotten.

As I summarize this section on love I have to clarify. When I talk about love, I'm not talking about some gushy fawning niceness; rather, love is something strong and silent that undergirds this gym. It is a kind of quiet ever-presence. It's connected to the camaraderie, the fairness, and the sequential focus on each individual. It supports the message that each person matters. Love makes this gym powerful.

Lead Spotter's Love, Summarized:

- Care about your guys.
- Give everyone a chance.
- Treat everyone fairly.

7. Heart

When I bench, I'm enthusiastic about pushing, but I am also conscious about getting done so the rotation goes quicker. The most awkward time for me is when I've gotten a breakthrough: a new number of reps or a new peak weight. The guys cheer me on and I get it. I don't know how to react. It's not my style to put my hands in the air and hop around. Instead, I quickly slink off the bench, and look sideways to try to make eye contact with one of the guys to acknowledge their support, then walk to the perimeter to wait for my next turn.

But one time, I got on the bench to lift. Dan trusted me with a big weight. I paused, and looked up at Dan and asked him to tell me that thing about *heart*, like I was asking my dad for a bedtime story. This is what he said:

> They say that all things can be measured: time, space, mass; but the heart of a man has no boundaries. How many times have you seen the impossible become possible?

I pressed the weight. I probably got a second rep in too. That's what gets me, *the heart of a man*. That's what makes me throw my notebook out the window: *The heart of a man*. That's what wins wars, crosses oceans, climbs mountains, and comes home again: *The heart of a man*.

Love is the greatest thing, but this chapter is about heart. Heart is not about what the gym gives the lifter, but what the lifter brings to the gym.

I wish I could define it, and I don't think I can trust the dictionary. The best I can do is to give a couple of examples, and apply this understanding to the Monstas who dwell in Dan's garage.

We made several references to lifting a car. It takes power, but we know darned well it also takes adrenaline. Prepping with a few years of squats couldn't hurt either. But it also takes heart.

I actually flipped a car once. I was driving North on the 15 with my wife. At the top of the hill near University Avenue the road used to slow down for traffic lights. We got there just as a car turned a corner too fast. I saw the white sedan roll several times into a vacant lot, kicking up dirt clouds. It landed upside down.

I pulled over and ran to help. By the time I got there, lots of guys were already pushing on the car. I slapped my hands onto the metal siding right by the rear door. As we pushed, gas gushed out in a thick stream all over me. I got scared and said "The gas . . .!" The guy next to me said, "Don't worry about the damn gas, just flip the car!" So, I had a lot of help. In fact, I wasn't much help at all.

What impressed me was the quickness of action of all the people who came out of the scenery to be part of the action. They got the job done without hesitation. That's heart.

Another manifestation of heart happened when my wife Paige gave birth to our first-born, Alex. Paige's mom and dad divorced and her dad died unexpectedly soon after. She was only six. Her family never gelled after that. She lived with her grandma, and then back with her mom. Her step-brothers and sister each left the house early, at about the age of 16. She lasted until she went to college.

When we came together and started a family, she wanted a real family, with lots of love. She took this attitude into that first childbirth.

When you see movies about babies you think they come out crying. In reality, if they don't cry, the doctor swats them on the butt to get them to cry so that their lungs clear. Then the babies settle down into a sleepy state next to the mom.

But that's not how it's supposed to go either. A baby might cry, but very soon after being born, he should stop crying and get absolutely quiet. He should open his eyes wide and look around the room, like a space alien landing on a new planet, taking in and processing the landscape around him. This is called the *quiet-alert* phase. Its main purpose is to let him learn what his mom looks like and start the bonding process.

The reason this doesn't happen so much anymore is that standard delivery procedures include drugging the mom at the base of the spine so she doesn't have to feel the incredible pain of childbirth. The problem is, it also drugs the baby.

Paige did not want her baby to be denied it's quiet-alert moments. That's love. When the pain started, this 22-year old girl did not give in, not even for a Tylenol. She endured it all, and got what she wanted. That's heart. She did the same thing for Cherish. She did the same thing for Jonathan.

If that's not enough heart for you, here's more. When I was a little kid, I saw a certain adventure film a couple of times. It's one of those oldies with pixilated monsters. The standard plot unfolded. The heroes were on some sort of quest to restore something that was lost. One by one they encountered witches, demons and monsters. One by one, guys got killed off till finally only one adventurer remained. When it looked like he was going to lose to the last monster, one of his former allies came back from the dead — by the sheer force of will — and assisted. That's heart!

Here's an example of no-heart. Back when I was a teenager working at Iron Man's Gym a guy came in. I thought he was a policeman, but Dan reminded me he was some sort of government agent. Regardless, most of these guys we encountered were strong. He was not. No big deal, he wanted a membership. We got him on a routine and we took him through workouts. Sometimes I took him. Sometimes Dan led him. But he never got strong. It never looked like he tried. We figure his bosses made him lift weights to get stronger, but his heart was not in it.

Flash forward to Monsta Gym — these guys want it. They want the power. But is it a worthy goal? Is it worth the investment of heart? It's just weights. It's just muscle. Yet, in addition to all the positive things I wrote about the value of power in the last chapter, this pursuit *does* have merit *because people want it.*

I have seen guys put their heart into lifts they previously thought they couldn't do. Each time they get it, they believe a little more. Their heart brings them that much closer to the next time, that much closer to that next amazing goal.

You have a goal; you matter. If it's important to you, you can apply heart. God put you on this earth. He has given you life. He has given you — as he has given each man — heart. Why half-ass through anything that's important? Use heart.

They say that all things can be measured: time, space, mass; but the heart of a man has no boundaries. How many times have you seen the impossible become possible?

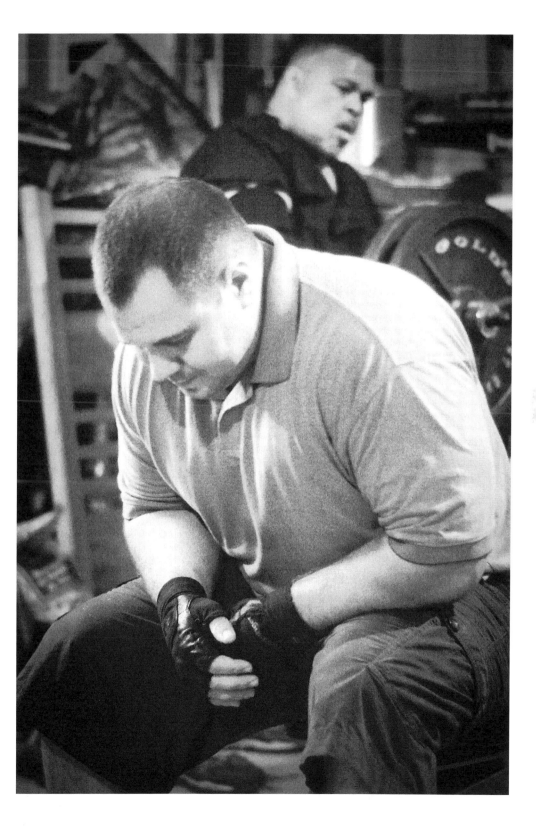

EPILOGUE

I decided to write about the Power Guru of Monsta Gym because I was impressed by the accomplishments. How could a place that trains so few guys result in five world records? I thought both the tale of the Guru and the How-to of the gym would be worth writing down.

I always thought about purity of application, seeing that the best possible outcomes would be for those men who started lifting in the gym and continued through their lives. And in reality, those are the guys who got the records. But what about those men who started somewhere else, and came to Monsta much later?

John Vaeena is one example. He is a local guy who heard of Monsta Gym, but never came by for a lift. He got impressively strong all on his own.

However, try as he might, he just could not break that barrier into the 300-pound club. That's when he came to Danny. That was six weeks ago. Now I see him at Monsta when I go up on Fridays, and he's repping 325 pounds.

I get to end with my story. I lifted 315 twice in my life, once at 19 and again at 24. Soon after I got married, I stopped lifting. When Alex entered high school fifteen years later, I started lifting with him. We got a weight set and put it on our back driveway.

I got pretty strong again. I was able to put on all the weights we had, barring one pair of 2 ½ pound-plates. I got 295, but I just could not get back to 300 pounds. I tried getting 300 by my 50th birthday. No dice, I got 295 two days later. So I thought I'd get it sometime during that year of life. Nope.

Just before I turned 51 I started going to Monsta Gym — finally. Dan and his brother Eddie both assured me I would get my goal, and then some.

Two months later I met Joe and our friend Michael at the Abbey in South Park. They hadn't seen me in a few weeks, and they were shocked at the growth in my upper body. But I still could not get 300.

I started to doubt my ability to get there. After all, I'm over fifty, so my testosterone has likely been on a glide-path down for a decade or two. Plus, as much as Dan said Monsta makes a difference, I know myself. I know I press hard every workout, and I am as consistent as a clock. I had also been doing some of the technique they do at Monsta, so really, if I've been working that hard for that long only to be sitting at an unchanging max, maybe I've found my limit.

Then, *last week* at Monsta I stepped up to the bar not really thinking much about it. There were two plates on each side. I got 10 reps. At Monsta, that's a warm-up. I'd never gotten that many at Monsta, or maybe anywhere. It seemed easy. When my time came around again, Dan was waiting with 285 pounds on the bar. I had gotten single reps with 285 at Monsta, but I fail at that weight as often as I get it. My goal for the night was to finally get a set of two reps with 285.

I got under the bar, and the first rep no longer had that slow painful bog-down one third of the way through the push. The second rep did, but I got it.

The next time around Dan was standing behind the bar with three plates on each side, 325 pounds. That's more than I ever lifted. I got under. Guys encouraged me. Dan told me to explode. It came down and I could visualize my pecs being stretched like nets under a trapeze artist. But those pecs pushed that bar all the way up without a stop. I finally got it. The next day I walked around the house feeling like a champion.

As I reflected on what kept me coming these past fifteen months I wondered if it was the 325-pound goal, the book, or the camaraderie. Well how about that? I got all three.

Printed in Great Britain
by Amazon